Praise for *Coaching for Caregivers*

"Yosaif August is the Vince Lombardi of coaching for caregivers."
—Andrew Schorr, two-time cancer patient; Author of *The Web-Savvy Patient,* Founder, PatientPower.info

"Yosaif August is quite the caregiving coach. His bee~ ~~~~~ -------- ------
ough compilation of resources for o~~~~~~~~~~~~~~~~~~~~~~~~~~~~~~~~~~
makes his book truly tremendous is h.
out for help, but on putting caregiver
—Hal Chapel, CEO and

"It's vital to take care of the caregiver! Yo.... uoes a terrific job of breaking down ways to do just that in a very consumable way."
—Sona Mehring, CaringBridge Founder and CEO

"I have been looking for a book on how to be a caregiver that is practical, accessible, concise and . . . gets them help where they decide they want it and need it. I have found it. This is also an excellent book for professional caregivers who coach family and friends and for the family and friends themselves."
—The Rev. George Handzo, BCC, CSSBB, Senior Consultant for Chaplaincy Care Leadership & Practice, HealthCare Chaplaincy, New York City

"Yosaif sure knows both coaching and caregiving, and his straight-forward and inviting style comes through loud and clear in his new book. The book should also be required reading for professional caregivers like doctors, nurses and hospice personnel."
—Ed Modell, most recent President of the International Coaching Federation

"If you're ready to show up for practice, Yosaif's coaching can help you and your loved one get the love and support you need."
—Bernie Siegel, MD, Author of *Love, Medicine and Miracles*; co-author with Yosaif, of *Help Me to Heal* (Hay House, 2003)

"If you want to buy a single book to help a family caregiver sustain herself or himself, this is it!"
—Roger J. Bulger, MD, FACP, FRCT; Retired, President, Assn. of Academic Medical Centers; Deputy Director, Center for Minority Health and Health Disparities, NIH

"Yosaif August's brief *Coaching for Caregivers* provides wisdom, practical solutions and practices and self-monitoring tools which can help generous, committed, giving persons to stay that way and to remain effective and engaged."

—Mack Lipkin, MD, Professor of Medicine, NYU School of Medicine; Director, Primary Care, NYU Medical Center

"The book encourages the reader to actually "reach out" for the support, wisdom, strength and love they need to continue in the role as caregiver. Written as if the author is speaking directly to you."

—Louise Knight, M.S.W., LCSW-C, OSW-C, Director, Family Patient and Family Services Program, Sidney Kimmel Comprehensive Cancer Center at Johns Hopkins

"Friends and family of caregivers should buy this book for them, look it over with them and help get them started in reaching out for the help they need."

—Daniel Wolfson, Executive Director, American Board of Internal Medicine Foundation

"It has always been CarePages' mission that no one go through a health event alone—including the ever-mighty caregiver."

—David Blanke and Krystin Reilly, *CarePages.com*

For additional testimonials, endorsements and reviews see:
www.yestolifecoaching.com/caregivers

In what concrete ways can your burdens be lightened?

In what ways would you especially appreciate being supported?

How can you share the care?

Come on inside . . . turn the page and let's get started!

COACHING

for

CAREGIVERS

How to **Reach Out** Before You **Burn Out**

YOSAIF AUGUST

QUICK COACHING TIPS SERIES: HELP WHEN YOU NEED IT

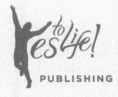

es life!
PUBLISHING

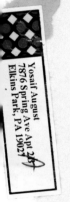

Ordering Information: Quantity sales. Special discounts are available on
quantity purchases by corporations, associations, and others. For details, contact the publisher at the address above.

Cover and interior design by Frame25 Productions
Cover art by Melpomene c/o Shutterstock.com
Author photo by Dion Ogust

US orders printed in the United States of America

Library of Congress Control Number: 2013936722
Publisher's Cataloging-in-Publication data
    August, Yosaif.
    Coaching for caregivers : how to reach out before you burn out / Yosaif August.
    p. cm.
    ISBN 978-0-9890626-1-9

    1. Caregivers—Psychology. 2. Caregivers—Family relationships. 3.
Adult children of aging parents—Family relationships. 4. Caregivers—Mental
health. 5. Children with disabilities—Family relationships. I. Title.

    HQ1063.6 .A95 2013
    646.7/8 --dc23
        2013936722

DISCLAIMER:
This guide is intended to provide guidance for caregivers to take care
of themselves. It is not intended to provide any clinical medical advice
or information, nor is it intended to be an alternative or substitute for
such professional medical attention. When facing a serious illness or
health condition, seek professional medical attention immediately.

HOW TO USE THIS GUIDE

To make best use of this guide when your time is precious, you may want to approach it in 10 minute reads. Start out by reading *A Note from Yosaif* and the *Introduction*, then scan the *Reach Out Roadmap* and the *Table of Contents*. Pick a topic that speaks to you and go right there. Find something immediate to think about or do. Do it. When the time or need arises, return to these pages to find other useful things to focus on – 10 minutes at a time.

REACH OUT ROADMAP

- Embrace the idea that this is the right time to reach out for love and support.

- Decide what you need.

- Take stock of your personal resources.

- Develop a positive and healthy mindset for your caregiving and discard beliefs that get in your way.

- Build on your strengths.

- Determine your privacy settings of boundaries and preferences.

- Identify your Inner Circle and let them organize themselves to help you.

- Choose the Reach Out strategies that make most sense to you.

- Let in the love that flows towards you.

- Be prepared for wondrous things to happen.

- Let people know how much you appreciate their love and support.

- Reflect with gratitude on all the blessings you have.

- Forgive, forgive, forgive yourself and others – over and over and over for being wonderfully human.

TABLE OF CONTENTS

PART TWO: REACH OUT (AND GET WHAT YOU NEED)

PART THREE: RESOURCES FOR REACHING OUT

To my dear sister Phyllis August-Rothman. For all the lessons about love, acceptance, connection, and kindness she is still helping me to learn. Thank God for Ground Hog day and our continual chances to get it right.

A NOTE FROM YOSAIF

Right now the idea of doing anything beyond what you're already managing to do may seem overwhelming. Even accepting love and support might feel like more than you're up to doing, let alone reaching out for it. Understandably, you may be just too worn out to even think about this.

Perhaps you're not quite that exhausted yet, but have noticed that you are getting more and more depleted as time goes on. And perhaps you can see that a very likely outcome, over the long term, is becoming drained by the weight you are carrying.

My intention is not to add another item to your to do list. Rather, it's to help you to hit the pause button for a few moments so you can begin a process to share the load and shorten your list.

We will focus on reaching out, not on burning out. I don't think you need to hear horror stories about what burning out can be like. Or see data about how caregiver burnout can impact your health, career, relationships, etc. If you are seeking that, simply Google "caregiver burnout."

I was motivated to write this guide in order to make your experience better than the one I had when I was managing my father's cancer care. I had been caregiving from afar until his medical needs required me to be with him for weeks at a time, hundreds of miles from his home and 1,000 miles from my own home, my family and the corporate consulting business my wife and I ran together.

Being at his side through all of this was some of the closest and most intimate time we'd ever spent together. And...I got burned out in the process. The cumulative effect of my caregiving was that I was so depleted, I developed a severe case of shingles.

I want you to take better care of yourself than I did. And reaching out for love and support, combined with other self-care practices, will help you do that. My goal for you is that you will be able to reach out easily for the help you need, when you need it and on the terms that feel good to you. You will be able to get the help you need without feeling intruded upon. I want to coach you to shed beliefs that may get in your way; to help you find ways of reaching out that respect your privacy and honor your values, personal preferences and needs.

I passionately believe that reaching out and letting the love flow in is some of the best medicine we can provide to our loved ones. It is also a sure fire way of avoiding caregiver burnout.

This is what I want for you. Acting through these pages as your coach, I offer the skills and understandings I have developed in my career as a life coach to help keep you going healthfully and resiliently. If even a single idea or technique here can lighten your load, I'll feel that writing this guide was worthwhile.

Take care, be well,

Yosaif

INTRODUCTION

Do you regularly help someone with rides to the doctor, provide meals, pay bills, help with bathing, grooming, dressing, walking or transferring to a wheelchair, take care of housekeeping, manage medications, arrange for outside services, and the like? If so, you, like 65 million other people in the United States and untold millions around the world, fill the role of caregiver. Moreover, while you may have chosen to become a caregiver, it is equally likely you have fallen into the role out of necessity, possibly without thinking about it or even recognizing it until well down the road.

Caregiving for someone can be very rewarding. It provides opportunities to demonstrate love and commitment, to experience deeper intimacy, to share special moments, and to live in harmony with spiritual and cultural beliefs. It can also be hard work. Caregiving can pose physical, mental and financial challenges to the caregiver. The tasks and responsibilities can be demanding, often involving sacrifices and competing responsibilities and priorities. Caregiving can disrupt relationships, threaten career opportunities and be a cause of mounting anger, frustration, guilt, anxiety, depression, and a sense of helplessness and exhaustion.

As the caregiver, at times you may feel alone, stressed and overwhelmed. Like so many others in your situation, you may be headed towards the common condition known as *caregiver burnout. Coaching for Caregivers* is designed to be the antidote, providing you with the essential tools you need to avoid becoming afflicted. It will show you how to take care of yourself while caring for another so you can healthfully sustain the help you are giving. And because as a caregiver you undoubtedly don't have time to waste, it will show you how to accomplish this in a concise, step-by-step manner, without a lot of fluff and filler. Think of it as having a coach by your side, guiding you to make choices and decisions that will help you to hold your life and that of your loved one in balance.

Coaching for Caregivers can be read straight through, or you can pick and choose particular sections to help you get through difficult moments. It will empower you to assess your needs, build upon your personal strengths, gather support, find outside resources, and more.

WHAT DEFINES A CAREGIVER?

You may be the spouse, significant other, son/daughter, intimate friend, relative, concerned neighbor or possibly even a paid aide of any of the following:

- Someone whose life may have changed in an instant, as with Cole Schlesner and his family, whose story appears below.

- Someone whose medical condition has emerged over time, as with Rabbi Arthur Waskow, whose story also appears below.

- Someone whose situation is chronic and will need continued care due to an ongoing ailment or the challenges of growing old, as with Ruth Rubin, whose story also appears below.

Perhaps you're in a sandwich generation where you are responsible for multiple people, including parents, spouse and children.

You may be living with the person whom you are caring for or nearby. Or, you may be looking after them from far away, managing the care provided locally by others and traveling to check in on them periodically. Each of these situations presents its own unique challenges and opportunities.

CAREGIVERS NEED CARE

Reaching out for love and support for yourself is fundamentally essential for you to have the physical, emotional and spiritual stamina to go the distance. *If you can say yes to most of these statements, this guide is for you:*

- I want to get the best care for my loved one.

- I need to make sure that the other areas of our lives continue to get handled.

- This is more than I feel I/we can handle by myself/ourselves.

- I know it will feel better to have loving support around us.

Perhaps you see the need for help but have been holding back from reaching out because:

- You are so stressed that the very act of reaching out feels like more time, energy and attention than you can spare.

- You feel like you are the only one who can do things for your loved one in the way they need to be done.

- You are afraid of becoming a burden to other people or of giving up your personal and family's privacy.

- You need support in learning how to ask for help or even who to ask it from.

- You know that reaching out is what you need to do. You simply need a nudge to do it.

HOW *COACHING FOR CAREGIVERS* WILL HELP YOU

If you haven't sought help for the above or similar reasons, PART ONE: REACH IN (BEFORE REACHING OUT) will help you get past these understandable barriers. It will:

- Help you clarify and prioritize the things you need now and may need in the weeks and months ahead.

- Help you tap your emotional and spiritual resources and build on your strengths.

- Inspire you to open up to receiving the love and support that is there for the asking.

- Show you how you can reap the huge benefits that reaching out can provide.

If you already recognize that you need help and are simply looking for ways to get it, PART TWO: REACH OUT (AND GET WHAT YOU NEED) will help you get moving. Choosing the smartest and avoiding the dumbest of the

Baker's Dozen Smartest and Dumbest Things You Can Do will help you start out on the right track. After these do's and don'ts are some practical suggestions about how to reach out in energy-conserving ways. They will:

- Guide you to mobilize your Healing Team - your Inner Circle and your Ever-Widening Circles of Support.

- Help you express your preferences about the way you'd like to receive support and set your privacy settings, i.e. how you'll maintain your privacy and personal space while opening up to loving care.

PART THREE: RESOURCES FOR REACHING OUT introduces you to the three major CARESITES and provides links to places where you can find information, resources and support. It also includes a Caregiver Self-Assessment Questionnaire, that you can use for taking stock of where you are right now. The section ends with a recap of the major ideas presented in this book.

Most sections start with a *Focus* that outlines the key topics in that section and end with *Reflecting and Acting,* helping you to apply what you've learned.

Along the way I offer *Coaching Tips,* which are like mini-coaching sessions on a particular topic. These reflect the co-active coaching approach I've been trained in. I avoid using coaching jargon, except when I use the term *gremlin* to call to attention those voices in our heads that sometimes pop up and tell us we can't do something we want and need to do. Since the purpose of this book is to coach you to reach out, my aim is to help you get past any gremlins that may get in your way.

Because I intend *Coaching for Caregivers* to be user-friendly and encourage you to make use of everything you already know, I've avoided using any medical or healthcare jargon or technical terms. However, I've coined a couple of new terms that I believe are helpful. I use the term PYCF for the *Person You Care For*, instead of the word patient, to distinguish it from the dictionary definition of patient as "submissive sufferer." PYCF emphasizes that it's a person—an empowered individual—we are speaking of, who inhabits the role of patient; it also speaks to the fact that this person happens to have a number of other roles in his or her life be they husband, wife, son, daughter, father, mother, sister, brother, friend, lover, partner, engineer, coach, comedian, surgeon, construction worker, etc., that the term patient seems to preclude or ignore.

I have also coined the term CARESITES to represent the user-friendly websites that people can use to gather love and support. The most prominent of these are *CarePages, Caring Bridge* and *Lotsa Helping Hands*. They are described in greater detail in PART TWO/Section VI: *Caresites*.

I know time is of the essence and you are eager to look at what you need right now: how to mobilize your strengths and resources and how to get rid of things that might be standing in the way of getting what you need. But first, I suggest you take a moment to be inspired by the stories of three families who were open to options that allowed them to head off caregiver burnout.

STUFF HAPPENS

It Happened in Loveland

Yes, believe it or not, Loveland is the name of the suburban town, on the outskirts of Cincinnati, where, on a balmy spring Sunday afternoon, in less time than a blink of an eye, the world changed for Cole Schlesner and his family. Their lives went from "perfect," as his father Scott describes it, to as scary as it can get.

Cole and his mom Wendy were at the baseball field at Stottman Park. It was Cole's day to pitch and she would be his good luck charm. And then the unspeakable happened. Excerpted from a posting on his CarePages site by his dad, Scott:

> "On Sunday May 17th, Cole was pitching for the Cincinnati STIX 14U baseball team, something he loved to do more than anything else in his life. Right after he released a pitch he was in a vulnerable position (still bent over) and a hard line-drive was hit back directly at him; the ball struck him in the head just above his hairline. He was originally conscious and coherent, but within 5-6 minutes Cole's condition dramatically changed and it became apparent he was seriously injured."

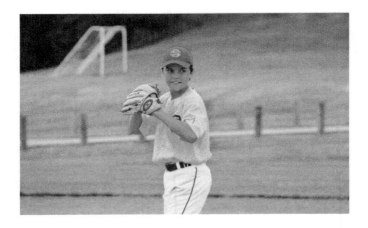

Cole was airlifted to Cincinnati Children's Hospital and diagnosed with a traumatic brain injury. He underwent emergency surgery and was then placed in an induced coma for three days. When he woke up he was paralyzed on his right side.

Over the next 45 days, Cole received rehab therapy in the hospital and continued with outpatient therapy for another year.

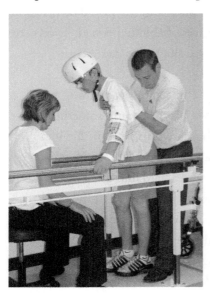

Cole was on track for recovery when, eight months post-injury, he began experiencing neuromuscular problems that affected his coordination and motor skills. He began having great difficulty walking, running and ultimately even speaking clearly. A neurologist described his condition as "one of the most rare and least understood diseases on the planet," and another specialist said it was "incurable." Since Cole had made such an extraordinary comeback from his original injury, this secondary setback was a much higher mountain to climb.

What helped the family all along Cole's three-year journey to recovery was the support they received when they reached out to their immediate community and through CarePages.

When Cole returned to school in the fall of 2011, he wore an orange bandanna to cover his shaved head and surgical scars. To his great surprise, he was welcomed by a huge outpouring of other students all wearing orange bandannas.

Through *CarePages*, thousands of people, including almost three thousand strangers, came forward to offer practical, everyday logistical help, from mowing their lawn, to helping with daily housework, to transporting their other three boys to all their activities. They prayed for Cole's recovery and continuously encouraged him during his treatments and rehabilitation. More amazing yet was that a group of family friends formed an organization called Play for 4 (Cole was #4), which raised thousands of dollars to help pay out-of-pocket medical

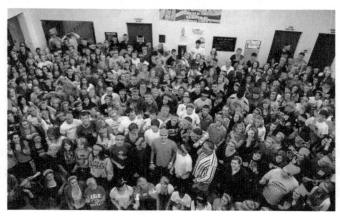

David Miller, *Loveland Magazine*

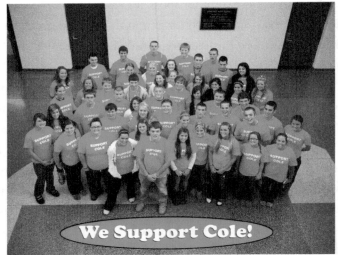

David Miller, *Loveland Magazine*

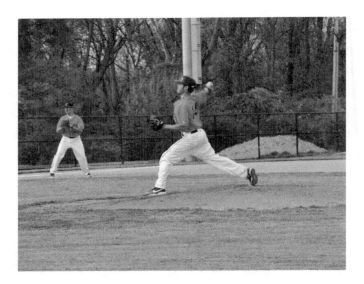

expenses for the Schlesners and also for other young athletes who suffered neurologic injuries while playing a sport. The organization even raised enough money to supply over 1,000 protective fielder's helmets for other young baseball pitchers.

In the Spring of 2012, Cole capped his astounding comeback with his return to the mound, striking out his first batter and getting a hit in his first time at bat.

This happy event was covered by a local TV station, which had been covering Cole's journey from the very beginning.

(See video link to *WKRC Channel 12 Cincinnati: http://www.local12.com/news/local/story/Back-On-The Mound/Wfok-dKjnXEK7w4hrMNwfog.cspx#.T23NpVAI8EU.facebook*).

Here's a recent photo of the Schlesner family.

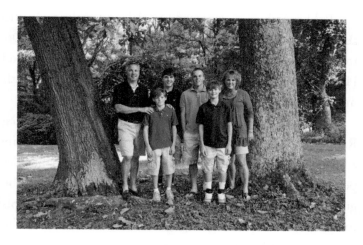

Stuff also happened in Mt. Airy, a small town-like section of Philadelphia, PA. It happened to Rabbi Arthur Ocean Waskow and his wife, Rabbi Phyllis Ocean Berman.

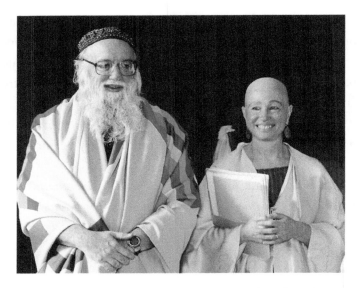

Rabbi Arthur, a renowned social and political justice advocate and writer, was being treated for throat cancer. Due to his radiation treatment, he was unable to swallow his food. His family feared he would die if he couldn't get nourishment. He reluctantly agreed to use a feeding tube.

But there were obstacles to making this happen. First, Rabbi Phyllis needed to learn how to do the feeding. During a visit to the home of close friends, she expressed her desperation about the situation. Appearing like an angel, another guest, a nurse she didn't even know, immediately stepped forward and offered to go right home with her to teach her how to do the feeding. It not only solved the how problem, it opened up the prospect that Rabbi Phyllis could, indeed, reach out to others for the help they needed.

The next challenge was logistical. Rabbi Phyllis commutes daily to her job in New York City and while she would be able to feed her husband before leaving for work and in the evening when she returned, he also required feeding in the middle of the day. They needed someone they could depend on to feed Rabbi Arthur every noon time. To find this help, she used an approach that today, ironically, could be considered old-fashioned. She simply reached out locally via the email list serves of three congregations in their community. Within a half hour, she had every day covered by volunteers. Surprisingly, most of the helpers were people she hardly knew.

This one act of reaching out saved Rabbi Arthur's life. Moreover, the people who showed up got an added bonus. The rabbi is a brilliant interpreter of the Torah, the Jewish holy book, and they got a chance to study with him during these noon time feeding sessions. Amongst them, they became what Rev. Dr. Martin Luther King called a "beloved community."

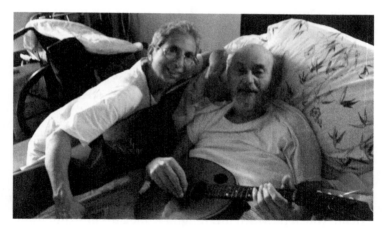

And then there is Ruth Rubin, whose story about caregiving and reaching out on behalf of her aging parents addresses a situation that more and more of us are facing. Ruth answered the call in particularly resourceful ways.

Ruth was the only child of Zeena and Ben. When Zeena became ill, Ruth moved from her home in Texas into their apartment in the Philadelphia area to care for them. Ben was 94 years old at the time and too blind and frail to care for Zeena himself. After 4 years, Zeena died and Ruth continued to care for her father.

In the process of caring for her father, Ruth took very good care of herself by reaching out for help that would prove to support them both.

When she reached out for hospice chaplaincy services, she established her own relationship with the chaplain, ensuring that she would also get the benefits of pastoral counseling. She arranged for them both to be on the chaplain's weekly schedule for home visits. She also reached out to the hospice's volunteer department and obtained a volunteer who visited weekly. During these visits, Ruth and the volunteer played Elizabethan music on the recorder together.

Ruth reached out to the VA to make sure that Ben got not only medical care and meds, but all the services he was entitled to: PT, OT, books on tape, music, eyesight evaluation, and more.

She reached out to friends via phone every day. She got their help and advice about personal and technical needs, especially about her computer.

She volunteered at the library every week, along with a friend, which provided meaningful work and companionship.

She also danced first thing every morning as a way of praying, dancing prayers of gratitude.

In the last years of Ben's life, Ruth began a daily practice of writing a poetic journal about her experiences as a caregiver. She wrote the last poem on the day Ben died.

When it came time let go of Ben's belongings, Ruth enlisted the help of a good friend and the services of a local company that helped with packing. Within two weeks, she was heading out west, onto her next journey in life.

The Schlesners used a CARESITE to reach out beyond their immediate circle. Rabbi Berman used the local congregations in her community to find support. Ruth Rubin utilized personal friendships and the services of local agencies. In each of these cases, they not only got way more than they needed, they were rewarded with way more than they expected. The help they received was material, emotional and spiritual; offerings that began on the physical level, e.g. delicious hot meals delivered to their homes, quickly and naturally evolved into emotional and spiritual support.

Helping helped the helpers, impacted their communities and sent ripples out to the wider world. Many helpers reported that their own life priorities and their way of viewing the world changed.

Your community may not be named Loveland, but there is undoubtedly an enormous amount of love to be harvested wherever you live. This guide can empower you, as caregiver, to receive the love, prayers and practical support you need as you navigate your way.

PART ONE

REACH IN
(BEFORE REACHING OUT)

Before you ask for help, you need to think about what kind of help would be most useful to you. Some people need practical help, others need someone to simply listen to them, while others need people to help maintain their spirit. Most people can benefit from all of these. If you are typical of many caregivers, you also may have trouble asking for the help you need. Which is why it is important to take a look at yourself before you do anything else.

1

YOUR NEEDS

What are your needs right now?

"When you know what you truly need, it's easy to ask for it."
—Rabbi Phyllis Berman

We'll Focus On . . .

No matter where we are in life, we all have needs in four areas: emotional, spiritual, mental, and practical. All of these areas need to be attended to during this time. Most of us would first and foremost focus on our practical needs – which are real, urgent and critically important. However, if you have these needs and haven't been reaching out, you've got some barriers to reaching out. And I think you'll find them and begin to get past them in the emotional, spiritual and mindset areas. So let's focus on them first.

Your emotional needs: In addition to coaching you to explore the kinds of emotional support that would be helpful to you right now, I will introduce you to a concept that might be new for you. I call it *trance*, which refers to the way we view the things that are going on in our lives. I will coach you to

3

develop ways of noticing when you're in such a state and how to snap out of an unhealthy and limiting one and move into one that is more open to possibilities.

Your spiritual needs: We will explore how to recognize and tend to your spiritual needs, even if the term spiritual is unfamiliar to you now.

Your mental needs: Given how much caregivers' stress relates to the inevitable uncertainties that come along, we will focus on the issue of uncertainty and how to manage it in the process of caregiving. I will coach you to create a Rolling Sense of Order, a technique you can use to manage uncertainty better.

Your practical needs: We will look at the things of everyday day life that you are handling which are currently more than you can healthfully handle.

YOUR EMOTIONAL NEEDS

Since this guide is about reaching out, what kind of emotional support would be helpful to you? Would you find having someone to talk to beneficial? Would you prefer someone who would listen unconditionally, or would you like someone who could also offer advice? Would this kind of support be better to get from a loved one or friend, or would it be more helpful to get some professional support, such as counseling or life coaching? Or would simply getting some snuggling time with your cat suffice?

What's going on for you emotionally right now? Are you so stressed that it seems like the very act of reaching out would take more time, energy and attention than you feel you can spare?

Do you feel like you are the only one who can do things for your loved one in the way they need to be done?

Are you reluctant to reach out because you are afraid of becoming a burden to other people or of giving up your personal and family's privacy?

Or, do you need some help in learning how to ask for help or even who to ask it from?

Wherever you are is where you are. And it's important and useful to recognize where you are and to do so without judging yourself. Usually these feelings contain some information that you would do well to take note of. It helps to ask yourself "what do I need to do right now?" Your choices are to move on or stay (stuck) with those feelings.

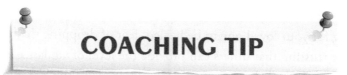

COACHING TIP

What Trance Are You In?

A term I often use to describe an emotional state of being is trance. When we're in a *trance*, we tend to see things in a particular way: delighted, calm, scary, hopeless, optimistic, edgy. Just as easy as it is to be in a grateful peaceful trance, we can all of a sudden find ourselves in a worried or panicked one. In times of stress and crisis, or even in times of exhaustion, the worried or panicked trance is often the dominant one. Once we notice that we are in a trance, we are no longer in it – unless we do things to prolong it. It's very much like when a hypnotist claps her hands to bring a subject out of a hypnotic trance.

As a caregiver, especially when you're dealing with the healthcare system, it's easy to fall into a trance of being confused, besieged, at war, prosecutorial, demanding, dominated, compliant, incompetent, and more. (You can surely come up with a few that are more familiar to you!) Since it's unlikely that someone will come along to clap their hands to snap you out of it, you'll have to find your own ways of doing so. And once you do, you're free to choose how you want to view the situation and how you want to act.

One more word for you as a caregiver in relation to the concept of trance: *martyr.* Martyrdom is possibly the easiest trance for caregivers to fall into and one of the most challenging ones to snap out of. This trance is induced by love, yearning for your loved one to be healed, fear of dropping the ball, not trusting that others can provide the level of vigilance and care that you believe only you can provide, and the like. Does this sound familiar? If so, it is understandable, but it is also untenable if you expect to be able to sustain your caregiving and remain reasonably healthy.

One of the goals of this guide is that you will be resilient enough to sustain your caring for as long as it is required. And that means finding ways to avoid falling into the martyr trance. Even Steve Jobs, the co-founder of Apple, who was a perfectionist and a control freak, learned to delegate. Otherwise he couldn't have built a successful company and made such a huge impact in the world.

COACHING TIP

How to snap yourself out of a martyr trance.

Begin by noticing if you have, at times, taken this martyr trance on. I think you'll know if it's true for you. If you're not sure, you may want to ask someone who cares about you for their perspective. When you are in a martyr state, reflect on what it feels like to be there. Notice how you are thinking, feeling or acting. Where do you feel the martyr in your body? Write down some words that could be a caption of a picture (or cartoon) of yourself during this time. You may even want to draw a picture to go with those words. What do you notice that can help you catch yourself when you're going into this trance? Is it a facial expression, a phrase, a feeling in your body?

Now, reflect on how you can snap yourself out of it and still be a loving, caring, dedicated caregiver. One way you might do this is to choose an image of someone you admire, such as a movie character, famous person, or someone you know, who would represent you as that dedicated caregiver. Then, as you notice yourself back in the trance, imagine that character handling the situation with more ease and spaciousness, and coaching you to follow them in doing the same. As you practice this, you will begin to discover that this is not only possible, but also a big relief for you.

Another way is one I call the iTunes/YouTube approach. I use songs to help snap me out of a trance at the moment

I notice I've fallen into it. They help me say yes to life. Try it out using songs you know or accessing them through iTunes or YouTube. For example, if you find yourself racing around frantically to ensure that every last thing gets done, try singing the phrase "slow down you move too fast" from Simon and Garfunkel's Fifty Ninth Street Bridge song. What might your song be: Theme from Rocky? A Little Help from My Friends? Puff, the Magic Dragon? Silly or serious, your chosen song will help you snap yourself back into a healthier and happier frame of mind.

YOUR SPIRITUAL NEEDS

To me, the spiritual realm is about meaning, purpose, values, ethics, and behavior. Many people find their spiritual lives nourished and supported within religious communities. Others follow spiritual paths and practices that are not associated with formal religions such as yoga and meditation.

Even if (or perhaps especially if) you wouldn't describe yourself as being spiritual, please don't overlook this section. It may speak to what is important to you, even though you might not use this language. If you aim at living a conscious life where you honor the values you consider important, that's what our discussion here is about. So please read on and feel free to substitute any alternative phrasing that works better for you than spiritual.

What are those needs right now? Take some time to reflect on what your spiritual challenges are and what questions are coming up for you. If you belong to a religious congregation or spiritual community and have an ongoing practice in your life, this may be a time to deepen or strengthen that practice. Or, it may be a time for you to reach out to members of your religious or spiritual community for help.

On the other hand, the notion of the spiritual dimension may feel unfamiliar or uncomfortable to you. Often challenging times, when we feel scared, unsettled, lonely, and adrift, can become times of spiritual awakening. This is especially so when we are dealing with a medical situation, when issues of suffering and life and death may come to the foreground. During these times you may feel that your usual ways of making sense of things aren't sufficient. If this rings true for you, ask people you know who have a religious or spiritual connection or practice to share with you how they access spiritual support in their lives. And be open to where this might take you.

YOUR MENTAL NEEDS

Let's take a brief moment to explore an important subject: uncertainty. Uncertainty is present in our lives from the moment we are conceived until we breathe out our last breath. (I guess the only certainty is that we will, indeed, at some point do that.) Ordinarily, we learn to live with and manage this uncertainty. We develop a working sense of order amidst the unpredictable things in our lives. We even get to enjoy some of this unpredictability. In so many ways, uncertainty is the spice of life: surprise birthday parties, unexpected wondrous moments, anticipation, suspense.

However, when uncertainty involves our health and well-being, our sense of control and orderliness can be shaken. And in trying to organize our caregiving activities, it can feel impossible to reach out for help because our needs are so unpredictable. Again, this can induce that martyr trance I've spoken about.

So how can you plan and organize your loved one's care amidst this unsettling unpredictability? The answer partly depends on whether you're in a critically acute situation or one that is stabilized and longer term, whether you're in the ER or ICU right now, or caring for a loved one with a chronic condition.

In most cases, we can create a sense of order even if the time frame is as brief as one hour. I call it a Rolling Sense of Order. I use the term Rolling Sense of Order because even as things keep changing, we can create some order in the moments in between these changes. Here's a coaching exercise to help you do this.

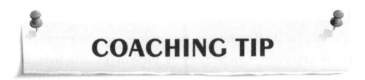

COACHING TIP

**How to live with uncertainty
by creating a Rolling Sense of Order.**

Choose an affirmation from the suggestions below or create your own about your commitment to your loved one and yourself. Reflect on it and either say it to yourself a number of times (with your eyes closed if you prefer) or write it several times on a piece of paper.

- I truly want what is best for my loved one

- My love and caring reflect my love

- I am lovingly taking care of my own well-being

- Love and caring are present for us right now

- I live happily and peacefully within the mysteries of my life

Consider what unit of time – an hour, day, week, month – seems most relevant right now. You may be in the ER waiting for a test result; you may be in the ICU waiting for a medical outcome; you may be at home tending to your loved one during their post-surgical recuperation. Ironically, even the uncertainty and unpredictability can have a predictability about it. For example, if you know that you won't know anything more for the next 24-48 hours because that's when your doctor will interpret some test results, that's a certainty that you can then use to create a temporary (rolling) sense of order. You can use this temporary order to organize what you need to take care of at this moment.

Given that time frame, what needs to get handled no matter what else happens? Choose one thing, even a small one, that someone else can step in and do. This might be taking your daughter to her karate lesson, being at your house to receive a package you're expecting, walking your dog, feeding your cat, or bringing some items or medications from your home. Thinking more spaciously, even in a time frame of a couple of hours you might consider getting a massage (and having the masseuse make a house call) or scheduling a life coaching session, which is easy to arrange since it is usually done on the phone or Skype.

Reach out for someone to handle some of the routine tasks. When you do this, you are developing your reaching out muscles. As you continue to do it, those muscles become both stronger and easier to use.

In the unpredictability of life, stuff happens. When it does, you can repeat this exercise. At times when you feel particularly stressed or overwhelmed, whether you do the whole exercise or not, remember your affirmations and then simply ask yourself what Rolling Sense of Order you can create at that moment. I think you'll be pleasantly surprised by the result as you regain your sense of control over things within your reach.

YOUR PRACTICAL NEEDS

Let's look at what's on your plate right now. What needs to be done? What must be done by you? *(see chart on the following page.)*

	FOOD	ERRANDS	BEDSIDE CARE	CHILD CARE	PET CARE	OTHER
MY NEEDS TODAY						
This Week						
Ongoing						
MY PARTNER'S NEEDS TODAY						
This Week						
Ongoing						
MY CHILDREN'S NEEDS TODAY						
This Week						
Ongoing						
PYCF NEEDS TODAY						
This Week						
Ongoing						
OTHER NEEDS						

REFLECTING AND ACTING

**Rate your current level of progress
(1 = low, 10 = high) in these areas:**

I am now more aware of being in a trance and have learned a technique to snap out of an unhealthy one.

1 10

I am clearer about my emotional, spiritual, mental, and practical needs.

1 10

I am familiar with the concept and technique of dealing with uncertainty by creating a Rolling Sense of Order.

1 10

Think about each learning outcome above and note 1) a new insight or understanding you've gained and 2) one thing you can do to immediately and easily apply it. Then, send yourself a one or two sentence email or text message to lock it in.

2

YOUR PERSONAL RESOURCES

This section will help you discover the significant emotional, spiritual, social, and logistical resources you can draw upon. You may well be surprised by what you find.

We'll Focus On . . .

- Beginning, continuing or renewing practices that promote the spiritual part of your life.

- Taking stock of your social and logistical resources and identifying new ones within reach.

- Enlisting your supporters to reach out to others on your behalf.

I know you have already developed your own unique ways of managing the emotional twists and turns of your life: how you embrace the joys and how you cope with the disappointments and tough things that happen. Whatever your way is, it's gotten you this far. Nonetheless, it pays to be open to finding new ways of seeing things that allow you to be more resilient, especially when there are bumps in the road, when people don't seem to live up to expectations or agreements, or when the medical system is not responsive to what your loved one needs at any given time. Noticing the trance you may be in, as I discussed above, is a new way you may want to try out.

As noted above, whatever your spiritual life may be like right now, however you access your inner support, this is the time to continue practices you have developed or to return to practices you know from the past are right for you. If you aren't familiar with a practice right now, ask people you respect where you might find easy access to some source of comfort, wisdom and inspiration. It could be something that you currently do but haven't seen as a spiritual practice, for example gardening, walking your dog, playing music, jogging, preparing a meal, or eating a meal slowly and, even better, silently. It may be a new concept to look into or a simple technique such as a meditation where you close your eyes and pay attention to your breath for a few minutes. You might think about attending a local yoga or mindfulness training program or joining a congregation or meditation group. I used a music compilation created for me by a friend in Gainesville and dubbed "Dr. Feelgood," each time I got back to my motel after a bedside visit to my dad. Alone in my room, I'd put on the tape and start moving and dancing to the music. At those moments, all that existed for me was the dancing and the music. With these practices, the spiritual aspect is less about what you do and more about the attitude and intention you bring to it.

COACHING TIP

Find a way for Dr. Feelgood to show up that is easy and natural and that you can do on a daily basis. For example, maybe that meal I referred to above, slow and perhaps silent, might serve you well. Once a day, take time for yourself, do nothing but focus on the experience of eating: taste, textures, temperature, aromas, things we so often miss out on when our eating becomes lost in our multitasking.

You can also create your own customized Dr. Feelgood musical experience. Make a list of five songs you'd love to hear when you need sustenance. Then think of five more. That's enough for a good-sized Dr. Feelgood album. If you know how to gather this music and put it on your mp3/tablet/smart phone/computer, or similar device, you're all set. If not, look for your nearest expert; these days it's often in the form of a ten-year-old who'd undoubtedly love to demonstrate what a breeze it is to do! Or you might try one of the new web-based music subscription services such as Pandora or Spotify.

As for social and logistical resources, most people have more potential practical help available to them than they initially realize. First there are your personal relationships, which might include family members, friends, organizations you belong to, co-workers, and your community at large.

Moving out from there are the many advocacy and support groups whose purpose is to provide assistance to people when they need it. This guide will help you find them (see Resources).

Among the most helpful resources are ongoing local support groups that embrace both caregivers and the PYCF. In addition to group meetings, they provide opportunities for you to discover new medical, financial, spiritual resources, and the like. In these settings, other caregivers share their secret shortcuts, strategies and personal network of contacts that they've developed to help along the way. You may also find a buddy to connect with, someone in a similar situation that you feel sympatico with. While there's no one exactly in your shoes, a buddy you make in a support group is probably the closest thing to it. Buddies listen, encourage, inspire, and can sometimes even conspire with you to take a little time off to treat yourselves to something special like a lunch out, a movie, a day at the spa… you get the picture! To help facilitate caregivers in finding buddies, the Kimmel Cancer Center in Philadelphia has recently added a Caregiver Buddy match program to their ongoing cancer patient buddy program. Of course, you needn't wait for your hospital to create such a program; go out and find the right buddy for you at one of these local group meetings.

Keep in mind that all your support doesn't have to be local. The team of caregivers for a friend in Philadelphia who used Lotsa Helping Hands and Caring Bridge had his website manager in Berkeley, California, his food coordinator in Boulder, Colorado, and the people who helped with logistics for moving and other tasks, in Philadelphia. He even had a coordinator in Sweden! These days the web is truly a world-wide web, in this case weaving together love and nurturance.

As you will learn in PART II, you don't have to investigate this all on your own. In fact, that is the point of making use of some of these resources.

COACHING TIP

You don't have to do all this reaching out yourself.

Allow people you know who are members of groups you do not belong to reach out on your behalf by tapping into their resources. For example, if you are not a member of a local congregation and have friends who are, they may be able to tap into their congregation's caring committee.

By using CARESITES, your supporters can sign up for tasks that will help you and not burden them. Using the help calendars they provide, enlisting people can be as simple and occasional or complex and frequent as they choose.

REFLECTING AND ACTING

Rate your current level of progress in these areas:

Starting, continuing or renewing practices that promote the spiritual part of your life

1 10

Taking stock of your social and logistical resources and identifying new ones within reach

1 10

Enlisting your supporters to reach out to others on your behalf

1 10

Think about each learning outcome above and note 1) a new insight or understanding you've gained and 2) one thing you can do to immediately and easily apply it. Send yourself a one or two sentence email or text message to lock it in.

3

YOUR PERSONAL STRENGTHS

||||||||||||||||||||||||||||||||||||||||||||||||||||||||||||||||||||||||||||||||||||||||||||||||||||||||||||||||||

We'll Focus On . . .

Here we will focus on revealing, appreciating and being able to access the strengths you currently bring to your caregiving.

||||||||||||||||||||||||||||||||||||||||||||||||||||||||||||||||||||||||||||||||||||||||||||||||||||||||||||||||||

This is another area where I'm certain you will be happily surprised. Whether you are in your teens or are a grandparent, your life experience has, in significant ways, prepared you for this moment. Let's take a look at what you bring to the table.

Let's first consider your personal strengths. This exercise will help you appreciate, value and access your strengths. Review the list below; add strengths that should be on your list or delete ones that don't belong there. Be prepared to add to this list as you go along. Ignoring some of your strengths is like ignoring a forgotten bank account that you've acquired along the way.

How would you rate your current level of comfort with each of the strengths listed below, as either OK or Need to Strengthen. As you add other strengths to this list, rate them, as well.

COACHING TIP

This is not necessarily a time for a major self-improvement project; be gentle with yourself as you do this .

	OK	NEED TO STRENGTHEN
Boundary Setting		
Assertiveness *Saying Yes* *Saying No*		
Clarity About What You Want/Need		
Sense of Humor		
Ability to Forgive (especially yourself!)		
Ability/Feeling Entitled to Recieve		
Allowing Yourself to Feel Vulnerable/Open		
Willingness to let go of judgments (again, especially of yourself!)		
Toughness		
Perseverance		
Resilience		
Courage		
Discernment		

COACHING TIP

This exercise will help you appreciate and access your strengths.

- Reflect on one of the items listed above, for example, resilience. Think of a time when you faced a tough challenging situation that really tested your ability to get through it.

- Now focus on how you were able to spring back afterwards, to get back to yourself. This may have taken a day or two or a good while longer. Focus on the fact that you had the inner strength to spring back, not how hard it was or how long it took.

- Think of another example or two of other situations where you also sprung back. That resilience is still within you in your core. You can access it any time you want, just like other things you've learned or skills you've developed in your life, such as riding a bike, swimming or using a keyboard (formerly known as typing!). To ensure that you lock in this memory and awareness of this strength of yours, you may want to write some notes or sketch a picture or download a Google image or a photo from your computer in a journal that you can refer back to. You can reinforce your access to that strength by periodically looking at that image or by simply noticing times when you are thinking about that strength. Doing so will easily and effortlessly move you in the right direction.

- *Optional*: Repeat this exercise with some of the other strengths listed above. You may want to do each one at a different time, allowing about five minutes each time. Don't make a chore out of this. Allow it to be as playful as you can. Let it be!

- *My prediction*: If you give yourself the time(s) to do this exercise and allow yourself to have fun with it – I especially enjoy the search for the right Google images or inspiring photos – you'll feel better and better about how prepared you are for what is in front of you. I'm so excited about your prospects that I'd love for you to share them with me at *august@yestolifecoaching.com*.

REFLECTING AND ACTING

Revealing, appreciating and accessing your strengths.

My strengths that I can comfortably access in my caregiving are:

My strengths that I was most surprised to discover are:

One area that I want to strengthen is:

Three possible ways of doing that are:

Of those ways, the one I've chosen to do is:

Send a quick email or text to yourself to lock these insights and commitments in.

4

YOUR BELIEFS

Developing a positive and
healthy mindset for your caregiving.

This section will help you commit to cultivating beliefs about reaching out for help that promote your well-being and that of your loved one, and to dispose of beliefs, or gremlins, that get in the way.

We'll Focus On . . .

- Assessing your readiness to reach out for what you need.

- Seeing if you suffer from RDD and, if so, some easy remedies for it.

- Using an *Entitlement Learner's Permit*, if you currently feel less than entitled to love and support.

- Choosing an affirmation that will help you to no longer need your learner's permit.

Let's get started. How do you feel about reaching out? What might be getting in your way?

Our beliefs can either support us in getting what we need or they can get in our way. This is especially important right now as you consider reaching out for the love and support you need. Reaching out calls for a willingness and a capacity to let go a little and allow others to shoulder some of the responsibility. This is not always easy to do. You can gauge your readiness by how you answer some of these questions about your personal feelings when it comes to asking for help in times of need.

1. People who ask for help are
   a) wimps
   b) self-indulgent
   c) wise
   d) misguided

2. If I reach out for support I will
   a) open up the floodgates and be overwhelmed
   b) open up the possibility of getting what I want and need
   c) undoubtedly be disappointed
   d) be wasting my precious time and energy

3. People I reach out to will mostly
   a) feel relieved to know how to be helpful
   b) consider me a pain in the butt and a burden
   c) feel uncomfortable and resentful
   d) be embarrassed

4. The right time for me to reach out is
    a) when things get a little easier
    b) when I have more on my plate than I feel I can handle
    c) any time that I feel it is the right time
    d) b and c

5. Some good reasons for reaching out are
    a) getting what I need when I need it
    b) having less burden on me and my loved ones
    c) giving people who care about me a chance to feel useful and not powerless
    d) a, b and c

6. By reaching out I can be sure that
    a) I will get unwanted advice and information
    b) I will have a better chance of getting what I want
    c) the wrong people will show up at the wrong times
    d) I will lose control of the situation

7. If I don't reach out
    a) the right people and support will simply show up
    b) I know I won't be disappointed
    c) I'll be stronger for having not done so
    d) I have less of a chance of getting what I need when and how I want it

8. Most people I would reach out to
    a) are way too busy and burdened already
    b) will appreciate knowing how they can help
    c) will be responding out of sense of guilt or obligation
    d) will be running as fast as they can to get away

9. After this situation is over
   a) I will owe people big time
   b) people will be appreciative for my letting them be there for me
   c) I will know that I really took care of myself and my loved one
   d) b and c

10. Asking for help makes me feel
    a) needy
    b) guilty
    c) empowered
    d) incompetent

11. When I'm really honest with myself about it
    a) I want to feel the love and support coming towards me
    b) I know people will appreciate the chance to help me
    c) I believe reaching out will relieve my loved ones and help them feel supported
    d) all of the above

Of course, there are no right answers when it comes to how you feel, but the following answers reflect the beliefs that support reaching out; other answers may reflect ways in which you may be holding yourself back from getting the support you need.

Answers: 1)c 2)b 3)a 4)d 5)d 6)b 7)d 8)b 9)d 10)c 11)d

A more in-depth discussion of the issues raised in this questionnaire can be found at *www.yestolifecoaching.com/caregivers*

COACHING TIP

Reflect on your responses to the above questions.

What immediate insights come to mind? How can these insights help you find your way during these challenging times?

What image or belief, whether it's one you've had or one which this exercise inspired, can really help you feel better, cope better, do better? What can you do to sustain it?

Which belief, or as I call it, gremlin, is calling out to be let go because it's getting in your way? What can you do now, today, tomorrow, and the next day, to discard it? Here are a few possible gremlin-removal strategies to consider:

- Change the internal station your mind is listening to, to one with an encouraging message. What might that better message say to you?

- Choose a song that brings that new message to life.

- Be playful with that gremlin – tease it, tickle it, play hide and seek, etc.

- Do some alchemy and change it into something wonderful. What can that be?

- What other things might you do?

A further note about our beliefs: Role models can often be helpful to us. But how many people do you know who are caregivers who are not on the road to burnout? People are often admired for how dedicated and self-sacrificing they are in taking care of their loved ones. But at what cost to their own health and well-being? We all want people to think of us as dedicated and able to do a good job, but there is a fine line between such dedication and martyrdom. Martyrs are known for many admirable qualities, but keeping their jobs and healthfully sustaining themselves so they can persevere are not necessarily among them.

Some caregivers are so sure that everything so depends on them that they never leave the house. No other family member or friend, no part time respite aide, no one (not even Dr. Oz!) can be entrusted with the mission of looking after their loved one. To leave the house would seem to be close to abandoning them. And surely, no one would ever want to do that. Granted this is a matter of degree and not a black and white situation, but if this in any way resembles your view of your situation, as Joan Rivers says, "can we talk?"

Let me be blunt. If you do burn out, in effect you will be abandoning your loved one. Thus you need to find ways, small ways, even tiny ways, to lighten your task and experience what delegating feels like. Can someone go to the drugstore to pick up meds or to the grocery for a carton of milk and a few other items that need to be replenished? Can someone return those library books for you and maybe look for another book by your favorite author?

Once you begin feeling more comfortable with this idea, explore other ways you can benefit from sharing the care. If your loved one is homebound, who could come over for an hour or two so you can go to the gym or out for a latte with a friend? With cell phones, it's easy to stay accessible in case you are needed for guidance or to return home sooner than you planned.

I'm so excited at the prospect of you doing this, that I would love you to tell me (*august@yestolifecoaching.com*) what steps you're taking and what the upside is for you and your loved one.

RDD: What is it?
What can you do about it?

Support can help you on your journey; isolation can make it a very arduous one.

Support helps when it's provided when we want it, in the ways we want it and when we are able to maintain our personal boundaries. Support helps the immune system. It also serves as a spiritual multivitamin. We know this because it feels so good.

But despite the fact that getting is as rewarding as giving, some people have a secret lingering condition, one that their closest intimates may not know of or are so used to they hardly notice it. I call it *RDD – Receiving Deficit Disorder*. Ask most people if they have an easier time giving or receiving and I'm willing to bet the more common answer is "giving, of course!"

If you suffer from RDD, and I really mean suffer, it means that no matter how generous you are with other people, somehow you just aren't comfortable receiving (love, care, gifts, praise) from them. The good news is, it's entirely curable. I recommend you try this simple twelve step program for overcoming RDD: All you have to do is reach out twelve times and let yourself receive what you're seeking and you're merrily on your way.

While that can work, you may have some beliefs that get in the way.

Some people think that reaching out is intrusive to other people. I guess it could be, under certain circumstances, but not most of the time. As you will discover, and so many of the Schlesner, Berman/Waskow and Ruth Rubin supporters found out, giving people a chance to make an immediate positive difference for you is a gift to them.

Some people think that reaching out demonstrates weakness. In reality, it is the other way around. It is a weakness to hold back from asking for what you need. Asking for what you need shows strength, even courage.

Some people hold back from reaching out because they feel they don't deserve it. As a life coach, my orientation is to help my clients get beyond their self-limiting beliefs by moving forward with action. So, for now, how about this practical advice from the twelve step programs, fake it 'til you make it. As a playful tool to implement this, I offer you an Entitlement Learner's Permit, a device Dr. Bernie Siegel and I developed for this purpose in *Help Me to Heal* (Hay House 2003). With blessings from Bernie and Hay House, here it is for you to use until you get the idea that you are naturally entitled and have thereby overcome your RDD.

Help Me To Heal ©2003 Siegel & August

ENTITLEMENT LEARNER'S PERMIT

This is to certify that _____ was born a totally and unconditionally lovable human being. Being aware of the imperfections humans may manifest, we nevertheless declare for all to acknowledge that _____ is entitled to be embraced with love, to be treated with respect and dignity, and to never have to apologize for asking for what he or she needs. This permit is valid until the aforementioned wakes up to the fact that such entitlement is his or her birthright.

_____

Bernie Siegel, M.D.,
Doctor of Unconditional Love

_____

Yosaif August,
Commissioner of Birthrights

COACHING TIP

Affirmations: An antidote to RDD

Affirmations are positive words; words are visualizations. The following affirmations can help you visualize yourself receiving the love and support you want and need during these challenging times. Try these out by writing them twenty times, or perhaps recording and listening back to them as you relax or while doing errands. You may find one or two that especially resonate for you or you may be inspired to write some others that work more powerfully. Post your favorites in a prominent place in your daily life (bathroom mirror, refrigerator, dashboard of your car, as a Post-it® on your desktop, etc.).

1. I love and deserve to be loved.

2. I show love for myself by taking good care of myself.

3. The more I open myself to receive, the more I can give.

4. Receiving love and support will help me keep going.

5. I owe it to myself and my loved one to take care of myself.

6. I show love for myself by opening up to love and support.

REFLECTING AND ACTING

Rate your current progress on developing a positive and healthy mindset for your caregiving:

Your readiness to reach out for what you need:

1 10

Identifying your beliefs that might get in the way of reaching out

1 10

Identifying your beliefs that support you getting what you need

1 10

Accepting your Entitlement Learner's Permit if you feel less than entitled to love and support

1 10

I don't need it; I already know I'm entitled! (check here)_____

Adopting one or more affirmations that will make it easier for you to reach out

1 10

The affirmation(s) I chose/created is/are:

Think about each learning outcome above and note 1) a new insight or understanding you've gained and 2) one thing you can do to immediately and easily apply it. Send yourself a one or two sentence email or text message to lock it in.

5

YOUR PRIVACY SETTINGS
Getting the help you need
without feeling intruded upon.

‖‖‖

We'll Focus On . . .

- Being able to say no as well as yes to help that is being offered.

- Feeling entitled and comfortable in setting your privacy settings.

- Identifying the most important privacy issues for you.

- Learning some tools you can use to do this.

‖‖‖

It's extremely important to set some boundaries and ground rules for how much privacy (physical, emotional, spiritual, as well as informational) you want. Think about how much you want to share outside your Inner Circle (the people who will be most intimately involved in your caregiving) and how you want it to be shared, e.g. updates on your CARESITE, through phone calls, in casual meetings between people. What are your preferences about how freely and with whom you want to talk about the medical condition of the PYCF, your own state of mind and other possibly personal issues?

COACHING TIP

Post a *Gone Fishin'* sign. Here's a powerful idea that can help you in managing the process of reaching out. Where reaching out is concerned, there is no such thing as a "point of no return." You and your Inner Circle can always post a Gone Fishin'sign, metaphoric or actual, on your hospital room, cubicle curtain, front door at home, CARESITE, voicemail message, list serve, etc., telling people who care about you that what you need most at that moment is rest, ease and privacy. You need to go Off Duty. You will let them know periodically how you are doing and if and when you'd like to resume actively connecting with them.

If you decide to set up a CARESITE, and I highly recommend that you consider doing so, your site will provide an easy place to let people know what you want, what you don't want, and when and how you prefer people to come forward. For example, you may ask people to check in with one of your Inner Circle people before making a hospital or home visit (both for the desirability of a visit and the possibility you'd like them to bring something or offer a ride to another person). You may also let them know if your loved one prefers brief and frequent visits to longer ones. Your CARESITE also offers privacy settings that allow you to decide who you want to be able to access your site – only people you specifically invite or anyone who hears about your situation and wants to reach out. Note: Stay tuned. There will be plenty of useful coaching tips for you and your visitors in an upcoming Quick Coaching Tips guide.

COACHING TIP

You can use the *Declaration of Interdependence* template on the next page or create your own to post on a CARESITE page or other mechanism you're using to let people know what support you need and how and when you need it.

PLEASE DON'T COME RIGHT NOW

Being able to say no is as important as being able to say yes. Knowing when to do each is where the gold is.

My dear friend Betsy sent me an urgent email: *"Mel is very ill and we do not expect him to live much longer."* I immediately booked a flight to San Francisco. Then I received a follow-up email: *"...so please don't come right now. Mel is just not wanting any visitors, even when he's alert and pain-free...it's too much for him. And I just want to come home at night, not talk to anyone, water the garden, and go to bed. Why don't I keep you up to date on his condition and we can see if there's a better time than now for you to come."*

Declaration of Interdependence

I feel so privileged to have you in my life right now and to know your intentions are aimed at my loved one's healing, comfort and well-being.

This statement will help ensure that the help and support you come forward with will be truly the kind of help we need, at the times we need it and in the ways we need it.

I don't expect you to read my mind about these things or to hold back in order to avoid being intrusive. My hope is that this statement will help everyone to be relaxed and feeling good.

First, the actions. We will be posting a daily notice of the things we need help with. Some will be daily, some for that week and some ongoing. They will be things I need, things my loved one needs, and things our family and household need done.

If you have time available, simply check this posting and either post your availability in the guest book or email or call whoever is listed for that task in the posting.

Now, my preferences for how I'm choosing to manage this journey.

ATTITUDES THAT WILL HELP US:
Positivity, honesty and openness
Please leave your worries on the doorstep

ADD YOUR OWN HERE:

_____

_____

BEHAVIORS THAT WILL HELP ME:
Ask me what I/we need right now rather than saying to let you know when we need something
Ask me if I want advice or information before offering it to me
Ask me if I want to discuss our medical situation at this time, please don't assume I do

ADD YOUR OWN HERE:

_____

_____

_____

Even amidst one of the most turbulent moments in her life, Betsy was able to hit the pause button and say no. She knew what she and her family needed right then and was able to say "please don't come right now." I cancelled my flight. Mel died the following week and I was invited to speak at his memorial service. It was the right time for me to be there.

You can read the entire story at my CarePages Quick Tips blog: *http://www.carepages.com/blogs/quicktips/posts*. In response to this blog, a reader shared how Betsy's action validated her own feelings. Her husband had been in a serious motorcycle accident and she was feeling overwhelmed by the outpouring of help. She was having trouble saying no, please don't come right now. "I was beginning to feel very wrong for pushing boundaries on even close friends and family. Thank you for your article. It made me feel normal vs. just grouchy all the time."

As you already read in YOUR NEEDS, wherever you are is where you are. It's important and useful to recognize this and to do so without judging yourself. It isn't about right or wrong. It's about what works for you!

One reader asked me for some guidance about how to say no. As I began writing a response, I realized quickly that this isn't really about yes or no. It's about opening up enough to get what you need without being so open that you feel intruded upon. It's about getting clear about what your boundaries are and being able to communicate them to the people who care about you.

This doesn't mean that doing so is truly easy. At first it can feel awkward. Or anxiety-producing. And there's no guarantee as to how your no will be received by the other person. They can be loving and gracious. They can be offended, even angry. You can only take responsibility for your side of the conversation.

That said, here are a few guidelines that can be helpful in eliciting the kind of response you are seeking:

Be clear, unapologetic and loving.

In her "please don't come right now" message to me, Betsy's explanation of what she needed (…I just want to come home at night, not talk to anyone, water the garden and go to bed…") and what Mel desired ("not wanting any visitors") was clear and unapologetic. Her suggestion, "Why don't I keep you up to date on his condition and we can see if there's a better time than now for you to come," was loving, as well.

Tell people what you want, as well as what you don't want.

For example, tell people it's best to contact you via email, but to not expect a response from you because you already have more than enough to handle. As described above, Betsy told me she didn't want me to visit at that moment, but she wanted me to be patient and wait for the appropriate time to do so.

Express your gratitude for their offering.

Whether or not you accept the help that is being offered, people need to know that you are receiving their offering of help, although perhaps not the actual help itself, as a gift to you that you value and appreciate.

Have compassion for others and for yourself.

Remember that you are doing the best that you can do right here and right now; it's not about doing the best that anyone could do in any circumstances anywhere. Likewise, so are the people who are coming forward to offer support. They are concerned and caring, but they may also feel awkward in not know how best to be helpful. A little bit of compassion for yourself and for them will go a long way.

Remember why you're doing this.

Your primary mission right now is to provide the best care for your loved one. Secondarily, but very close to primarily, your mission is to take the best care of yourself. Reaching out supports both of these missions.

Forgive, forgive, forgive. Yourself and others.

REFLECTING AND ACTING

Getting the help you need without feeling intruded upon.

Rate your current level of progress in these areas:

I feel it's okay for me to set my own boundaries as I reach out for help.

1 10

I am comfortable in doing so.

1 10

I am comfortable with my ability to say no when my needs require it.

1 10

The main privacy issues for me are (list some):

I am familiar with tools I can use.

1 10

The tool(s) I'm most likely to use is/are:

Think about each learning outcome above and note 1) a new insight or understanding you've gained and 2) one thing you can do to immediately and easily apply it. Send yourself a one or two sentence email or text message to lock it in.

6

BENEFITS

||||||||||||||||||||||||||||||||||||||||||||||||||||||||||||||||||||||||||||||||||||||||||||||||||||||||||||||||

We'll Focus On . . .

Our focus here is on the benefits reaching out brings to you, your loved one and those you reach out to.

||||||||||||||||||||||||||||||||||||||||||||||||||||||||||||||||||||||||||||||||||||||||||||||||||||||||||||||||

From my own experience, as a PYCF, a caregiver and a member of an Inner Circle, opening up to receiving love and support from other people has so many things to recommend it:

- It feels good.

- You feel loved and valued.

- You can find comfort.

- You can get emotional and spiritual support.

- It helps you feel connected and reminds you that you're not alone.

- You get things you need.

45

- You get things you want, including things you didn't even realize you wanted.

- You get better access to medical information and resources.

- Your family gets taken care of.

- The PYCF gets supported.

- You feel the energy of the prayers and healing wishes people are offering on your loved one's behalf.

- You get some great meals and snacks.

- You can take a break and tend to your own needs.

- You can connect with and learn from other families dealing with similar issues and situations.

- You and your loved one get help with the important logistical things that keep your lives going.

In PART TWO, Section VI, CARESITES, you will read the wisdom that families have shared with me to encourage you to follow their example in reaching out. Meanwhile, note that people who your reach out to (and those others who also care about your loved one who reach out to you on their own initiative) get abundant immediate benefits:

- It simply feels good to be of help.

- It helps lower their anxiety by allowing them to be actively involved in doing something useful. It's empowering and deeply satisfying for them to have a chance to make a difference for your loved one.

- It helps lower their frustration at not being able to otherwise impact your loved one's medical situation.

• They get an endorphin flow.

Also, by using a CARESITE, you give other caregivers a chance to get the satisfaction of being able to help others beyond their own loved one, which is a gift to them. It also can help take their mind off their own troubles.

REFLECTING AND ACTING

Reflect on what your own list of benefits might look like.

In what concrete ways can your burdens be lightened?

In what ways would you especially appreciate being supported? For example, would having someone simply listen to you non-judgmentally be useful?

TAKE A MOMENT NOW....

Now that you have done some personal reflection, you might want to take a little time before moving on.

Hit the pause button.

Relax.

Notice your breath.

Let yourself do nothing for a while. Don't TRY. Just let yourself be.

Once you've cleared your mind, take stock of what you have done so far.

- You've had a chance to look at the range of needs you and your loved one have – practical, emotional, mental, and spiritual.

- You may have noticed beliefs that have held you back from getting your needs met and begun to shape a new attitude about doing so.

- You may have looked at your strengths and personal resources and seen new possibilities for using them.

- And, I hope you've considered the importance of being able to establish your own privacy settings in order to freely reach out without concern about being intruded upon.

There's only one right way to have done this – your way. Consider this a work in progress; later on you may periodically return to any of the topics in Part One and do some more exploration or simply to appreciate how much awareness and effectiveness you have attained along the way.

Now it is time to enter the next phase, PART TWO: REACH OUT (AND GET WHAT YOU NEED). It begins with some advice from experienced caregivers about how to approach reaching out in a positive way. It then presents some useful concepts and strategies for reaching out.

As you go forth, I offer a playful paradox: How to reach out without it becoming another item on your "to do" list. Analogies that come to mind: considering what to order from a restaurant menu with many tasty options; surfing with your TV remote for just the right program for a particular moment; deciding which birthday present to open first. With the information you find in the following pages, reaching out will hopefully become as routine as grabbing the remote and settling down for a much needed respite.

So, hit the resume button, turn the page and begin to REACH OUT.

PART TWO

REACH OUT
(AND GET WHAT YOU NEED)

Now that you have taken stock of your needs and can see the huge benefits you will gain by reaching out, you are ready to focus on how to accomplish this most effectively and efficiently.

BE SMART

The baker's dozen smartest/dumbest things to do when reaching out

To start, let's focus on some advice that some very resilient caregivers have shared with me.

Do these smartest things:

1. Get clear about what you want and need.

2. Get clear about the way you want people to offer help and support.

3. Set your privacy settings; let people know your limits, boundaries.

4. Tell people up front if you are not comfortable talking about the medical condition of the PYCF in order to honor his/her wishes for privacy.

5. Let people know your overall medical/healing goal for the PYCF.

6. Understand that people will react differently to your news and unexpected people will rise to the occasion, while others you thought would be there may fade away.

7. Forgive people in advance for their clumsiness, awkwardness, unconsciousness, and stupidity.

8. Forgive people for not showing up. It's not about you, it's about them and the other things going on in their lives.

9. Create a designated team captain.

10. Know that solo is dodo.

11. Realize that only you are in your shoes; no one else knows what you are experiencing and need unless you tell them.

12. Let people know how they can best speak to the PYCF about her/his medical condition and care.

13. Let people know that you prefer them to directly ask you how they can help, e.g. "what can I do for you right now or this week," rather than "let me know when you need me to do something for you."

Avoid doing these dumbest things:

1. Assume it's best for you to tough it out alone.

2. Assume that other people know what you need.

3. Focus on not hurting other people's feelings.

4. Be afraid of asking too much of other people.

5. Think that asking for support shows weakness on your part.

6. Take help and support on any terms people offer it.

7. Take other people's lack of help as a personal affront.

8. Assume you must let go of your personal privacy and boundaries during this time.

9. Feel like you have to suffer fools.

10. Let people wear you down with unwanted information and advice.

11. Assume that by opening up to support, you have to be open with everyone.

12. Think that only you can get everything done correctly.

13. Assume that you won't get burned out later, because you're able to handle things well now.

REFLECTING AND ACTING

Which of the smartest things resonated most for you?

Which of the smartest things will be a challenge or a stretch for you?

Which of the dumbest things gave you a new insight into what you need to do or avoid doing?

GATHER YOUR CIRCLES OF SUPPORT

We'll Focus On . . .

Who you will reach out to, either directly or through other people. *We'll look at:*

- Who to include in your Inner Circle of support

- Your options for reaching out to your Ever-Widening Circle of Support

---

YOUR INNER CIRCLE

Your Inner Circle consists of the people who will be most intimately involved in your caregiving. This group of people will be the prime movers when it comes to organizing others to extend your circle of support into your Ever-Widening Circle of Support. Who will you invite into your Inner Circle?

__ spouse/partner/ significant other

__ parents

__ children

__ brothers/sisters

__ other relatives

__ friends

__ neighbors

__ co-workers

__ clergy

__ members of organizations you belong to

__ clinical professionals

__ other professionals (spiritual advisors, non-traditional health practitioners, healthcare advocates, etc.)

Whether you, the PYCF or someone else is the ringleader, the PYCF must always be in the center of the Inner Circle, setting the direction, making the decisions and calling as many of the shots as they want to and are capable of. As their condition changes, their involvement may change, as well.

Each member of your Inner Circle can take the lead in a particular area of care: food, household chores, visiting schedules, errands, bringing things to and from the hospital, medical research, setting up and managing your CARESITE, team captain, and the like. Some of them may be part of your medical decision-making process. You can appoint someone as the orchestrator/choreographer of your Inner Circle. They can have some fun by being playful and creative in casting people in the roles you need, i.e. court jester, bouncer, announcer, diplomat, PR person, and so on.

As you move forward on your journey, the most important rule is to pay attention to what the PYCF, you and perhaps other members of your household need at each point along the way. More is only better if more is what you want and need.

Something else to keep in mind is the well-being of your Inner Circle and how they can balance the other parts of their lives with being actively engaged in caring for the PYCF and supporting you. They, too, may need physical and mental/spiritual relief. You certainly don't want to see your helpers burn out or feel overburdened, so be sure to check in with them and give them a chance to tell you when they are feeling overwhelmed or simply cannot be available. Your Inner Circle may be like a tag team where some members need to leave and find replacements to pass the baton on to. When you are stressed, it can be hard to remember their needs. And, of course, whenever you can, express your appreciation.

YOUR EVER-WIDENING CIRCLE

Your Ever-Widening Circle of Support consists of the people that your Inner Circle will reach out to for broader community engagement. You have several options to choose from to generate this next level of support. You can:

- Have an Inner Circle person create a simple email list serve to keep people informed and let others know what you need and when and how you need it.

- Use the existing list serve of your congregation or other organization you are actively involved in, including Yahoo and Facebook groups. Also, as suggested above, you can extend the circle of support by asking people to tap into their own networks, which you may not be a part of.

- Create a CARESITE (see Section V, below).

- Create and use a Facebook page.

- Reach out to a peer support group (see RESOURCES).

- Hire professional home care or respite care.

REFLECTING AND ACTING

Gathering your Circles of Support.

Make a list of everyone you have invited into your Inner Circle and define some roles they can each play:

Create your Ever-Widening Circle, choosing amongst the alternatives listed above that are easiest and most available to you. Make a list of who can help get you started using one or more of these options or help you find more information.

3

CAREGIVING FROM AFAR

We'll Focus On . . .

The focus here is on caregiving from afar, which is becoming commonplace as more and more of us are being called upon to provide caregiving for aging relatives who don't live nearby. This might mean assisting a sibling or other family member who lives closer and provides most of the onsite caregiving or care managing, or you might be the primary caregiver, taking on the task from a distance.

Caregiving from afar generally involves finding and hiring the right services and managing them remotely. You may be dealing with medical professionals, social services, health insurance companies, and more. You may also be managing your loved one's finances.

I was the primary caregiver for my parents, who were living in Florida, while I lived in New York. My sister lived in Jerusalem. After my father died, my mother moved to an assisted living facility. My sister came in from Jerusalem for an extended visit, chose the facility with our mother and helped her to move in. I hired an aide who was working there to assist my mother with her medications and personal care. I hired a bookkeeper to pay her bills and another service to file health insurance claims. Ultimately, I hired a care manager, too. And while she was in a post-stroke rehab facility, because she loved music and loved to sing, I hired a music therapist to visit her a few times a week. (The facility actually hired a music therapist later after they saw how good it was for my mother.)

I monitored her care by speaking with her daily and making periodic trips to Florida. All these services worked well, except the personal care aide. On a visit, I noticed that my mother's teeth were terribly chipped. The aide claimed to have no knowledge of how that happened. I was appalled. If the aide hadn't noticed it, that was neglect; if she had noticed it and ignored it, that was worse. And, if she had somehow been responsible for it…. I fired her and hired another aide who turned out to be an angel of love and compassion. But this was an example of one of the challenges of managing care from afar and reinforces the importance of creating a local team you can trust. (One night I got a call from the aide. She had accompanied my mother to the ER. She enabled me to speak with my mother directly, calm her down and help reassure her that things would be okay. What a blessing to have this aide on our team.)

One note of caution. Be security conscious in terms of your loved one's valuables. Earlier, with my father's in-home care, we weren't so careful and some things seemed to have vanished.

If you are caregiving from far away, among the professional services to consider hiring is a care manager, a professional trained to find and manage a range of services, especially for elders. You can find such people by using the resources listed in PART THREE of this guide.

You will also find CARESITES a great way to get emotional, spiritual, practical, and logistical support. If your siblings, other relatives and friends are spread out all over the country (or world), a CARESITE will help you all to keep in touch and involved with what's going on.

Caregiving from afar may an unavoidable option and not being able to directly ensure that proper care is being provided can, itself, be a cause of considerable stress. If so, you will be doing your best if you also attend to your own well-being. If you've skipped PART ONE of this guide, I urge you to go back and see which topics speak to you.

COACHING TIP

A feel-good exercise to help you appreciate yourself for all you're doing.

This ten-minute exercise will clarify what is truly important to you and help you feel better about your caregiving whether it's been done from nearby or from afar. And, caregiving from afar may be the best you can do right now. However without unlimited time, money and other resources, and with other demands on your time and attention, you may feel understandably frustrated. Let's focus not on these limits, but instead on what is truly important to you.

First, take a few moments to relax and center your attention on your breathing. Simply watch your breathing; don't try to control it. Now, think of a time in the future, maybe a year or two from now. Put yourself in a place you'd like to be. From that place, look back to the present time and to the caregiving you are providing right now. Do this with an appreciative eye. Be careful not to discount things that seem obvious, expected or no big deal. Include things that you may actually resent doing or may be doing out of a sense of guilt or obligation. Make a list of these things. Then look at each item on your list and reflect on what about doing that task is important to you, or what value of yours you honor by doing it. Write these down next to each action. Again, with an appreciative eye, see what these tell you about the importance and worthiness of what you're doing right now. With that in mind, write an email to yourself from your future self that you visualized before, thanking yourself for honoring those values. Send it. Receive It. Believe it. Read it again when you need it .

REFLECTING AND ACTING

If you are caregiving from afar, make a list of the local people you have assembled to help the PYCF with daily needs.

How satisfied are you with this team you have created ?

1 10

What changes do you want or need to make?

How did the self-appreciation exercise work for you? Did any gremlins show up, i.e. voices saying things like "you're not doing enough" or "if you were a good son/daughter you'd be..."

Think about each learning outcome above and note 1) a new insight or understanding you've gained and 2) one thing you can do to immediately and easily apply it. Send yourself a one or two sentence email or text message to lock it in.

4

GETTING IN SYNC WITH YOUR MEDICAL TEAM

~~~~~~

We'll Focus On . . .

Your medical team is one of the most critical focal points. We'll focus here on how you can communicate effectively with doctors, nurses and other medical professionals so that your loved one gets the best care from them and that your interactions with them don't contribute to your burn out.

~~~~~~

The patient-and-family-centered approach to medical care, which is becoming the norm these days, calls for the person being cared for, the caregiver and the medical professionals to work together. With this approach, the PYCF, alone or through you as the caregiver, is the decider—the most important person in the decision making process. And your clinical providers are essential to helping her/him make the best decisions. Unfortunately, conversations with clinicians can be challenging. Since it is your loved one's life, and the quality of that life at stake here, learning to interact effectively with your medical team is crucial.

The medical people working with the PYCF can be an enormously helpful resource to you as the caregiver, but the process of interacting with them can also create a huge source of stress. As we explored earlier, uncertainty and ambiguity can present a daunting challenge when you're dealing with a medical condition and can clearly be a cause of caregiver burnout. One way of minimizing this is to ensure that you are kept informed as much as possible and can trust that this is the case.

Here are a few suggestions for how to best interact with doctors, nurses and other medical professionals.

GETTING PERMISSION

First and foremost is to get permission in writing from the PYCF for each of the medical people involved to discuss the PYCF's medical condition with you and have you included in treatment decisions.

CLARITY: GETTING IT RIGHT

Being informed requires that clinicians explain medical issues in ways that you can understand. This is essential in order for you to participate in decisions that need to be made.

It may be helpful to paraphrase what you hear and confirm that is what your physician actually means. If you are at all unsure, ask for a translation into terms that make sense to you. In recent years, medical schools have been giving more attention to teaching physicians to do this more effectively.

It may be helpful to make an audio recording of these conversations, with their permission, of course. Listening to the recording when you're more relaxed can be very helpful to your understanding or for raising additional questions you may have. Another approach is to bring someone along with you whenever possible to provide another pair of ears.

ACCESSIBILITY: REACHING YOUR DOCTOR WHEN YOU NEED TO

Ask each of your health care providers how they prefer to communicate with you and come up with a way that works for everyone. Ask them for the best language for you to use to indicate your urgency when leaving a message, for example, "request," "priority," "highest priority." You may want to come to an agreement on the response time to your request calls or emails. For simple requests, you may arrange for a response within a day or two. For more urgent issues ("priority," "highest priority") you may need a quicker response. Find out from them how to best indicate how quickly you need a response. Understand that the demands on their time are unpredictable, but preparing in this way can help mitigate problems.

COORDINATION: MANAGING YOUR CARE

Enlist one person, preferably the primary care doctor or specialist who is directing the care of the PYCF, to coordinate with the other medical professionals who are part of the care team and to interact directly with the PYCF or you, as their surrogate and point person. Their coordination should include consulting with each other as appropriate, keeping each other updated and ensuring that they all have access to the most recent medical records. Don't assume that this coordination is happening. Periodically, ask the primary physician which clinicians she is in touch with, whether the latest lab test results are being shared with other physicians involved and how recent this contact has been. Doing this respectfully once or twice will let your doctor know you're on top of things and expect her/him to be as well. This is another place where a little effort can go a long way.

An increasingly useful way of being in the loop is to have access to an electronic records system. These are just coming online now, so check with your provider to see what is available and to explain how to use it. If they don't have one, you can set up your own electronic personal health record (PHR). See *www.yestolifecoaching.com/caregivers* for a list of recommended providers.

REFLECTING AND ACTING

Is your medical team part of your circle of support?

How ready are you to work out an agreement with your medical and other providers?

1 10

What barriers, if any, do you have in working with the medical team?

Are any gremlins lurking in the shadows telling you to mind your own business or other things that would put you out of the loop? If so, what message are you're hearing? (For some gremlin removal strategies, see the Coaching Tip that follows the self-assessment questionnaire in the PART ONE: YOUR BELIEFS. If you are feeling intimidated, go back and fill out your *Entitlement Learner's Permit* as described in that section.)

If you're having trouble communicating or understanding the medical situation, pick someone in your Inner Circle to assist you. Beyond the three areas discussed above (clarity, accessibility and coordination), what other concerns do you and your loved one have in working with your medical providers?

Think about each learning outcome above and note 1) a new insight or understanding you've gained and 2) one thing you can do to immediately and easily apply it. Send yourself a one or two sentence email or text message to lock it in.

5

CAREGIVING DURING TRANSITIONS FROM THE HOSPITAL OR REHAB

llllllllllllllllllllllllllllllllllllllllllllllllllllllllllllllllllllllllllllllllllllllllllllll

We'll Focus On . . .

The focus here is on change, as the PYCF moves from one setting to another.

llllllllllllllllllllllllllllllllllllllllllllllllllllllllllllllllllllllllllllllllllllllllllllll

Many hospitals still refer to the process of releasing patients as discharging them. What an image! Like being fired out of a cannon. In *Help Me to Heal*, Bernie Siegel and I offered a new term. We said that empowered patients and families are *encharged*.

Family caregivers often find transitions home, whether they mark the beginning of caregiving or happen after extended periods of caregiving, to be times of heightened stress and anxiety. This is for good reason. Caregivers often feel ill-prepared to handle the follow-up medical procedures, as Rabbi Phyllis Berman sensed about her ability to utilize the equipment for feeding her husband Arthur. Studies recently found that 20 percent of Medicare patients are readmitted to the hospital within thirty days. And 40-50 percent of those are avoidable. However, they have also found that when continuity and coordination of care, accuracy of post-hospital medications and post-hospitalization home care are managed well, and when there is collaboration with community resources for support, people are much less likely to develop the problems that put them back in the hospital.

Because these issues are being given a great deal of attention by hospitals and medical providers these days, in part due to the enormous costs involved when people are readmitted to the hospital, the language has begun to change and evolve into what are called "transitions in care." As such, your hospital may offer the support of a transitional care specialist or transition coach who can, at least temporarily, be a valuable participant in your support team.

If the hospital or rehab doesn't offer transitional care support, find out how you can go about getting it. Hint: Start with the facility's social work department, and look for people with such titles as care manager, nurse navigator or discharge planner. Two excellent resource links are caretransitions.org and NTOCC.org. Also, see PART THREE: RESOURCES.

Another change that may be happening is that your loved one may be experiencing a chronic condition or may now be in a different phase of such a condition. If this is the case, then your caregiving also needs to transition into what is now called "chronic care management." Learning about and embracing the concepts of this kind of care will enable you to be empowered and proactive in helping your loved one get what she/he needs. The reaching out to do here is to the professional caregivers in the facilities you've been dealing with.

REFLECTING AND ACTING:

When it comes to caregiving during transitions from hospital or rehab, to what degree do you feel prepared to do what you need to do?

1 10

What information do you need?

What kinds of advice or guidance would be helpful?

Who in your Inner Circle or other resourceful person could help you find these resources?

Think about each learning outcome above and note 1) a new insight or understanding you've gained and 2) one thing you can do to immediately and easily apply it. Send yourself a one or two sentence email or text message to lock it in.

6

FINAL COACHING TIPS

You're well on your way towards finding your own ways of reaching out and avoiding burning out.

You've looked at your needs, strengths, beliefs, personal resources and more. You've been introduced to some concepts and strategies to help you to reach out.

The following section, PART THREE: RESOURCES FOR CAREGIVERS provides you with powerful tools and resources for you to use. I will introduce you to the three major CARESITES and show you how easy they are to set up and use. You'll hear from some very wise family caregivers about the many ways these CARESITES helped them and how you can reap the same benefits for you and your loved one.

There's a list of caregiver resource directories that are easily accessible to you on the web and a list of organizations that provide a wide range of supportive resources for you to tap into.

My own website (*yestolifecoaching.com/caregivers*) also provides continually updated links to other caregiver resources, including links to videos of some of the families featured this book.

Meanwhile, I offer you some final

COACHING TIPS

- Embrace the idea that this is the right time to reach out for love and support. It is there waiting to be called forth.

- Let in the love that flows towards you.

- Appreciate the wonderful opportunity you are providing to people who are extending themselves to you.

- Be prepared for wondrous things to happen.

- Let people know how much you appreciate their love and support.

- Reflect with gratitude on all the blessings you have.

- Forgive, forgive, forgive—yourself and others—over and over and over for being wonderfully human.

PART THREE

RESOURCES FOR REACHING OUT

1

CARESITES

Choose them and use them.

We'll Focus On . . .

CARESITES are free, easily created and user-friendly websites you can use to gather love and support.

The three main CARESITES that thousands of people are now using are the focus of this section. They are:

www.carepages.com

www.lotsahelpinghands.com

www.caringbridge.com

||||||||||||||||||||||||||||||||||||||||||||||||||||||||||||||||||||||||||||||||||||||||||||||||||||||||||||||||||||||||||||||||||||

All of the CARESITES above provide simple online instructions to set up your own site. Each one also provides privacy settings that, as we've mentioned before, allow you to let in love and support while ensuring that your privacy concerns are respected. I recommend you review each site's privacy policies so you are aware of how they use the data they collect.

Before you decide to set up a CARESITE, visit each one in order to choose one, or a combination, that feels right to you.

The following are screen shots of the home pages and tools for the three CARESITES.

CarePages

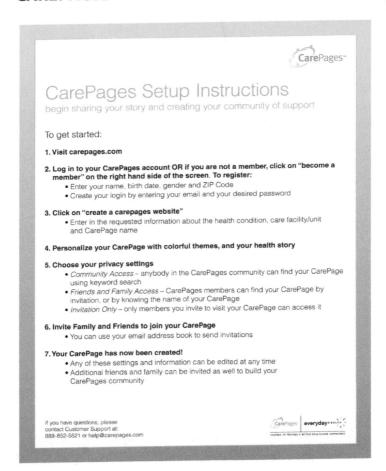

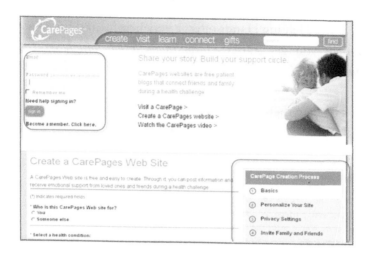

LOTSA HELPING HANDS

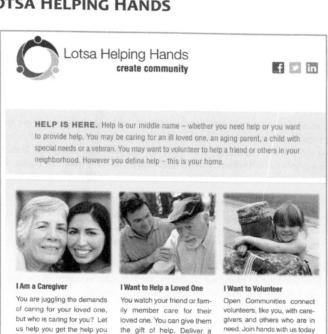

Lotsa Helping Hands
create community

HELP IS HERE. Help is our middle name – whether you need help or you want to provide help. You may be caring for an ill loved one, an aging parent, a child with special needs or a veteran. You may want to volunteer to help a friend or others in your neighborhood. However you define help – this is your home.

I Am a Caregiver

You are juggling the demands of caring for your loved one, but who is caring for you? Let us help you get the help you need.

I Want to Help a Loved One

You watch your friend or family member care for their loved one. You can give them the gift of help. Deliver a meal, organize visits, provide what they need so that they can care for their loved one.

I Want to Volunteer

Open Communities connect volunteers, like you, with caregivers and others who are in need. Join hands with us today through one of our Open Communities and help us care for those in need.

Lotsa Helping Hands offers a very helpful and brief video to help you get started: *https://www.lotsahelpinghands.com/ how-it-works/*

Here are their step-by-step instructions:

Ready to get started? Let's go.

1. Click on the 'Get Started' tab
In minutes, you, a friend, or a family member can fill out the form on this page. Simply enter the name of the Community being created and your name and email address. Who should create the Community?

2. Make a list of what helpers can do
Go to the 'Administration' tab in your Community and begin posting volunteer needs with our easy-to-use templates. For instance, this might include dinner on Monday, Wednesday and Friday nights or rides to medical appointments on Tuesday mornings. When a new need is posted, everyone in your Community will get an email. The system also sends reminders to volunteers with the time, date and activity of their commitments.

3. Invite the people who want to help
Next, enter the names and email addresses of those you wish to be part of your Community. Start with people who have expressed interest in helping. You can add more people anytime. No one can join your Community unless they are specifically invited by you. Those whose names you entered will receive a welcome message that will explain the service and give them all the information they need to easily join in and get started.

4. Grow your community as you go
As you like, you can add more to your Community — post photos, create custom sections, add resources from our nonprofit partners and more. Community Members can join in by posting well wishes, sharing announcements and sending messages to the family.

5. Watch our Getting Started Webinar
Learn how to create a Community of support: the first steps in setting up the Help Calendar and inviting Members to your Lotsa Helping Hands Community.

Here's an example of an actual Lotsa Helping Hands home page:

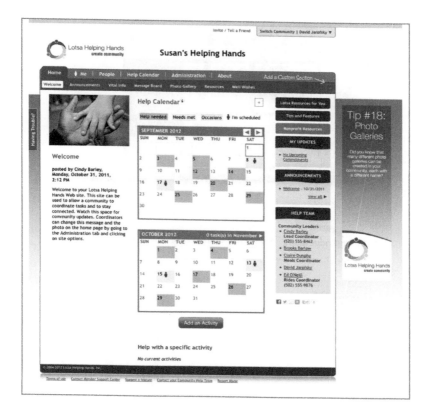

As you can see, Lotsa Helping Hands (above) and Caring Bridge (below) provide very useful calendars where people can post things they need or need done and visitors can directly sign up for them. These allow people the chance to be helpful and to do so in increments that suit the other needs and demands of their lives. You can easily use these calendars in conjunction with CarePages or with list serves.

CARING BRIDGE

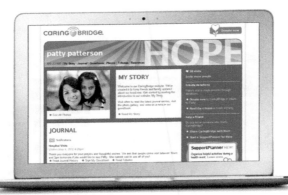

CaringBridge .org *Connecting Family and Friends When Health Matters Most*

Support Home > Find An Answer > How do I create my own CaringBridge website?

Search by Keyword	Search

Personal CaringBridge websites are not searchable. Find out more

How do I create my own CaringBridge website?

To create a CaringBridge website for yourself, just follow these steps:

Step 1: Get Started

1. Connect to www.caringbridge.org.

2. On the left side of the page, click the **'Create a Site'** button.

3. Click the circle next to **'Myself'** and enter your e-mail address.

   Please note: The First and Last Name fields will not be clickable. You do not need to enter this information when creating a site for yourself.

4. **Check** box next to, "*I am at least 18 years of age AND have read and agree to the Terms of Use.*"

5. Click purple **'Preview Website'** button.

Step 2: Log In/Sign Up

- If you are logged in to CaringBridge, you will skip directly to Step 3.
- If your e-mail address is registered with Caringbridge, you will be asked to enter your password and click **'Log In.'**
- If you have not registered before, please follow the website's prompts to create a profile with your First and Last name and a personal password you will use to log in with. Then click the purple **'Sign Up'** button.

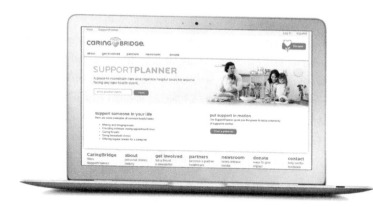

CARESITES can be the Rolls Royce of reaching out. If you need more convincing, here are some quotes from some very wise, experienced families, super-users of CarePages, who agreed to let me share them with you. As a result of using CarePages, they gathered an Ever Widening Circle of thousands of people, many of whom started out as strangers. You can reap these benefits with any of the CARESITES discussed above.

Using CARESITES to reach out provides an easy, efficient way of keeping people updated about what is going on.

"The three main benefits for us were chronicling our experience, sharing it with others, and receiving support through the messages."

"It provided instant access to any and all friends and family wanting to know how Andrew was doing, taking the daily burden of returning calls and emails off of us, his primary caregivers."

CARESITES let people know what you need logistically, emotionally and spiritually.

"Once we realized that our journey was going to be a lot longer than we initially thought, we used CarePages to ask for help. It was very useful in getting a request out and allowing people to help. For example, with me living in the hospital full time and Justin working, we needed extra help with our older son Matthew. He was in nursery school at the time but that was not every day. Friends and neighbors jumped in to help care for him on off days and after school."

CARESITES connect you with other families dealing with similar medical conditions.

"It allowed us to search for other families with the same disease, providing a support system immediately. HLH is rare and until Andrew was diagnosed, we had never heard of it or knew anyone else with it."

"Using CarePages search tools, other cancer parents found me and, in turn, I found other cancer parents. It was so nice to find others who understood, who could share insight, who could offer hope."

"CarePages has made it easier to find others affected by the same disease and be able to make connections to these families. To know that you are not alone is vital in this journey. I can honestly say the support system we developed from having Liam's CarePage carried us through some very difficult times."

CARESITES provide you with an emotional outlet.

"CarePages provided us the ability to voice all of our feelings without being interrupted or judged. We shared our fears, worries, frustration, sadness, and anger, as well as our joys, small victories, insights, and blessings."

"For me, it was also a way to clear out the intensity of the day so I could start 'fresh' in the morning. I think writing is a little like a pressure valve, releasing some of the stress. It also forces you to put your thoughts in order and make sense of it before hitting 'post' and purging it from your mind."

"CarePages was my public journal, allowing me a place to vent, to share my thoughts and feelings. Being the parent of a sick child is stressful and often lonely. CarePages helped me to feel more connected."

CARESITES open up a channel for you to receive love and support.

"In the morning I would awake to the uplifting messages of love and support that my friends and family would write in response. I would share many of the comments with my daughter. It was like taking a vitamin that helped get us through the day. We felt surrounded by the ones we loved even though we were not only physically distant, but necessarily isolated much of the time."

"Of course the messages of support and encouragement throughout our journey were priceless. There were countless days that the only highlight was getting to read the messages on our CP. It was amazing to see how many friends and strangers alike were following our story and praying for us."

"Above all, you learn a lot about people, some family and friends and others strangers, from the messages left on our page. When you live out of a hospital room day and night and for 6 months straight, having the CarePage to turn to is priceless. I can't tell you how many nights I stayed up reading others'

CarePages, looking for some comfort or information. I looked forward to all the messages that would come pouring in. The support is priceless."

"Everyone needs a soft place to land—a place that they can feel at home, comfortable, content. When going through a rare, terrible, complex illness, be it yourself or a family member, that place can be difficult to find."

CARESITES help you help others. ·

"Through our sons' experiences we have learned a lot and have become advocates for many things. The importance of joining the National Marrow Donor Program, as well as being a regular blood donor. We have used our CarePage to educate and encourage others to do so as well."

"We never wanted for a book, a toy, toiletries, or anything. Sometimes we would use the CarePage to request general donations for others. I also use it still to post current information about upcoming events for CHOP (Children's Hospital of Philadelphia) or Sara's Smiles (the foundation we set up)."

"We also shared photos of happy times and painful times. We wanted to raise awareness about childhood cancer, to show how long and difficult the road is for the child and family."

CARESITES help you to stay in touch.

"CarePages helped me reconnect with old friends, strengthen current friendships, and make new friends."

CARESITES empower people who love you to do things that are useful for you and to get past their sense of powerlessness to otherwise change the situation you are in.

"It helps people feel good about themselves since they know they are helping you and know you welcome their help."

CARESITES provide a way of keeping a record of the caregiving journey

"CarePages served as a medical record. I was able to go back through entries to see when procedures were done, when phases began/ended, what meds were used, if Ali had any reactions, etc."

2

OTHER RESOURCES
FOR REACHING OUT

Visit our website, *http://www.yestolifecoaching.com/caregivers*, where we periodically update the list of resources for caregivers. Also, as you discover other valuable resource listings, let me know (*august@yestolifecoaching.com*) so we can add them to our website and to updated versions of this Guide.

THE FOLLOWING ORGANIZATIONS HAVE EXTENSIVE RESOURCE LISTINGS AND LINKS

Rosalynn Carter Institute for Caregiving:
http://www.rosalynncarter.org/caregiver_resources/

National Alliance for Caregiving: (301) 718-8444
http://www.caregiving.org/resources

Caregiving Action Network: (800) 896-3650
http://caregiveraction.org/resources/

Lotsa Helping Hands:
http://www.lotsahelpinghands.com/
resources/#resources-from-non-profit-partners

Patient Empowerment Network:
http://www.powerfulpatients.org/wp/
Patient Power: *http://www.patientpower.info/*

Well Spouse Association: *http://www.wellspouse.org/resources*

Family Caregiver Alliance: (415) 434-3388
www.caregiver.org

Medicare Hotline: (800) 633-4227
www.medicare.gov

National Information Center for Children and Youth with
Disabilities: (800) 695-0285
www.nichcy.org

211: Dialing 2-1-1 will provide you with free and confiden-
tial information and referrals for help with food, housing,
employment, health care, counseling, and more. To see if
there is a 211 service in your area, go to *http://www.211.org.*

CAREGIVING RESOURCES

National Alliance for Caregiving
4720 Montgomery Lane, 5th Floor, Bethesda, MD 20814
www.caregiving.org, info@caregiving.org

Today's Caregiver Magazine
Family Caregiver Alliance (FCA)
180 Montgomery Street, Suite 1100, San Francisco, CA
94104
(800) 445-8106
www.nahc.org/Consumer/coninfo.html or
www.caregiver.org, info@caregiver.org

Caregiving Action Network
10400 Connecticut Avenue, Suite 500 Kensington, MD
20895-3944
(800) 896-3650 or (301) 942-6430
http://caregiveraction.org

Family Caregiving 101
www.familycaregiving101.org

Well Spouse Association
63 West Main Street, Suite H, Freehold, NJ 07728
(800) 838-0879
www.wellspouse.org, info@wellspouse.org

Children of Aging Parents (CAPS)
P.O.Box 167 Richboro, PA 18954
(800) 227-7294
www.caps4caregivers.org, info@caps4caregivers.org

Next Step in Care
http://www.nextstepincare.org

CAREGIVING FOR VETERANS

National Caregivers of Veterans Support Hotline:
(855) 260-3274
www.caregiver.va.gov

Guide to Long Term Care for Veterans
http://www.va.gov/GERIATRICS/Guide/LongTermCare/index.asp
(http://www.va.gov/GERIATRICS/Guide/LongTermCare/
Shared_Decision_Making.asp)

Veteran's Caregiver Self-Assessment Tool
*http://va.gov/GERIATRICS/Guide/LongTermCare/Caregiver_*
Self_Assessment.pdf

RESPITE CARE

National Adult Day Services Association, Inc.
85 South Washington, Suite 316, Seattle, WA 981 04
(877) 745-1440
www.nadsa.org, info@nadsa.org

ARCH National Respite Network/
National Respite Locator Service
800 Eastowne Dr. Suite 105 Chapel Hill, NC 27514
(919)490-5577
www.archrespite.org
Includes the National Respite Locator, a service to help caregivers and professionals locate respite services in their community.

AGING RESOURCES

AARP

601 E Street, NW, Washington, DC 20049

(888) 0UR-AARP (687-2277)

www.aarp.org

Care for the caregivers Web page:

http://www.aarp.org/home-family/caregiving/
care-for-the-caregiver/

Eldercare Locator (to find local services)

(800) 677-1116

www.eldercare.gov

National Association of Professional Geriatric Care
Managers

3275 West Ina Road, Suite 130 Tucson, AZ 85741-2198

(520) 881-8008

www.caremanager.org

TRANSITIONS IN CARE

Care Transitions

http://www.caretransitions.org

Survival Skills for Leaving the Hospital:

http://www.caretransitions.org/caregiver_resources.asp

National Transitions of Care Coalition

http://www.NTOCC.org

HOSPICE

Hospice Foundation of America
1710 Rhode Island Ave, NW Suite 400, Washington, DC
20036
(800) 854-3402
www.hospicefoundation.org
haoffice@hospicefoundation.org

Hospice Net
www.hospicenet.org/html/caregivers.html

National Hospice & Palliative Care Organization (NHPCO)
1731 King Street, Suite 100, Alexandria, VA 22314
(800) 658-8898
www.nhpco.org

CAREGIVER SELF-ASSESSMENT QUESTIONNAIRE

Caregiver self-assessment questionnaire
How are YOU?

Caregivers are often so concerned with caring for their relative's needs that they lose sight of their own well-being. Please take just a moment to answer the following questions. Once you have answered the questions, turn the page to do a self-evaluation.

During the past week or so, I have ...

1. Had trouble keeping my mind on what I was doing .... ☐ Yes ☐ No

2. Felt that I couldn't leave my relative alone .... ☐ Yes ☐ No

3. Had difficulty making decisions .... ☐ Yes ☐ No

4. Felt completely overwhelmed ..... ☐ Yes ☐ No

5. Felt useful and needed .... ☐ Yes ☐ No

6. Felt lonely............................... ☐ Yes ☐ No

7. Been upset that my relative has changed so much from his/her former self .... ☐ Yes ☐ No

8. Felt a loss of privacy and/or personal time .... ☐ Yes ☐ No

9. Been edgy or irritable............... ☐ Yes ☐ No

10. Had sleep disturbed because of caring for my relative .... ☐ Yes ☐ No

11. Had a crying spell(s) .... ☐ Yes ☐ No

12. Felt strained between work and family responsibilities .... ☐ Yes ☐ No

13. Had back pain .... ☐ Yes ☐ No

14. Felt ill *(headaches, stomach problems or common cold)*........... ☐ Yes ☐ No

15. Been satisfied with the support my family has given me........... ☐ Yes ☐ No

16. Found my relative's living situation to be inconvenient or a barrier to care .... ☐ Yes ☐ No

17. On a scale of 1 to 10, with 1 being "not stressful" to 10 being "extremely stressful," please rate your current level of stress. _____

18. On a scale of 1 to 10, with 1 being "very healthy" to 10 being "very ill," please rate your current health compared to what it was this time last year. _____

Comments:
(Please feel free to comment or provide feedback.)

AMA
AMERICAN
MEDICAL
ASSOCIATION

Self-evaluation

To determine the score:

1. Reverse score questions 5 and 15.
   (For example, a "No" response should be counted as "Yes" and a "Yes" response should be counted as "No.")
2. Total the number of "yes" responses.

To interpret the score

Chances are that you are experiencing a high degree of distress:

- If you answered "Yes" to either or both questions 4 and 11; or
- If your total "Yes" score = 10 or more; or
- If your score on question 17 is 6 or higher; or
- If your score on question 18 is 6 or higher

Next steps

- Consider seeing a doctor for a check-up for yourself
- Consider having some relief from caregiving (Discuss with the doctor or a social worker the resources available in your community.)
- Consider joining a support group

Valuable resources for caregivers

Eldercare Locator
(a national directory of community services)
(800) 677-1116
www.eldercare.gov

Family Caregiver Alliance
(415) 434-3388
www.caregiver.org

Medicare Hotline
(800) 633-4227
www.medicare.gov

National Alliance for Caregiving
(301) 718-8444
www.caregiving.org

National Family Caregivers Association
(800) 896-3650
www.nfcacares.org

National Information Center for Children and Youth with Disabilities
(800) 695-0285
www.nichcy.org

Local resources and contacts:

SIA-08-0011-PDF-1-08

4

RECAP: REACH OUT ROADMAP

Embrace the idea that this is the right time to reach out for love and support. It is there waiting to be called forth.

Decide what you need. List the kinds of support and concrete help you need and when you need it.

Take stock of your personal resources, in particular those resources you already have and "low hanging fruit," i.e those that can be easily accessed.

Develop a positive and healthy mindset for your caregiving and discard beliefs that get in your way.

Build on your strengths. Take an inventory of personal strengths that you bring to your current challenges. Commit yourself to appreciating these strengths and also to noticing when you are getting stronger and more effective in an area that is important to you and your loved one.

Set your privacy settings of boundaries and preferences. This will ensure that you get the help you need without feeling intruded upon.

Identify your Inner Circle and let them organize themselves to help you. Tell them what you want and how you want to get it and let them coordinate things. You may want to receive your active support from your Inner Circle only and have them keep your Ever-Widening Circle updated.

Choose the Reach Out strategies that make most sense to you. Select one or more of the following to keep people informed and let them know your needs and how to fulfill them:

- Use the existing list serve of an organization that you are actively involved in.

- Create an email list serve of people you want to be in touch with. You can manage this yourself, but it may be less stressful to have an Inner Circle person take charge of the emails.

- Create a CARESITE.

- Set up a Facebook page.

- Join a support group.

Let in the love that flows towards you. Appreciate the wonderful opportunity you are providing to people who are extending themselves to you.

Be prepared for wondrous things to happen.

Let people know how much you appreciate their love and support.

Reflect with gratitude on all the blessings you have.

Forgive, forgive, forgive—yourself and others—over and over and over for being wonderfully human.

ACKNOWLEDGMENTS

First, I want to thank Gene Schwartz ("Mr. Gene"), long-time devoted friend, mentor, cheerleader, business consultant, and surrogate father, for his wise advice that led me to create this series of *Quick Coaching Tips Guides*.

I also appreciate Bill Gladstone, of Waterside Productions, for his encouragement and support. It's great to have Bill in my corner.

Nikki Goldbeck, my tried, true and wise editor, has helped to shape this guide in ways large and small, with deep wisdom and humor, from the very beginning. Along the way, she has also served as my coach and mother confessor. Thanks, also, to her dear husband, David, for recommending her editing services to me. I also want to thank Ellen Frankel, for her early support in shaping this project.

I want to thank Bernie Siegel, MD (aka Dr. Bugsy Siegel), my *Help Me to Heal* co-author, for the ongoing loving support and friendship he has extended to me over the past twenty or so years.

My gratitude also goes to the good folks at Hay House, my valued publisher, especially Donna Abate, who directs Hay House's *Heal Your Life* blog (*www.healyourlife.com*), who has so generously encouraged my writing and blogging. (See *www. healyourlife.com/search?q=yosaif* for my articles on the blog.)

I am so grateful to Jonathan Friedman of Frame25 Productions for his brilliant design work that has so well brought this book to life and for Matthew Friedman for bringing *Yes to Life!* to life!

I am very grateful to Wendy and Cole Schlesner, Rabbi's Arthur Ocean Waskow and Phyllis Ocean Berman, and Ruth Rubin for how generous they've been with their time, wisdom and resources. Special thanks to the Schlesner and Berman-Waskow families for their permission to use their family photos in this book.

I want to thank CarePages/Everyday Health, especially David Blanke, for immediately supporting my vision for this series and reaching out on my behalf to their CarePages super-user families, those whose CARESITES grew to hundreds and thousands of caring people. Also Elyse Beasley for inviting me to write my *CarePages* blog (*www.carepages.com/blogs/quicktips/posts*) and the following *CarePage* managers who generously shared their wisdom with me: Kristin Akin, Alicia Ambroso, Karen Borgen, Jennifer Burke, Mark Carlinsky, Beth De La Cruz, Alexis g., Ida M. Hall, Stephanie Jacobson, Jon Levin, Michelle Schulze, and Melissa Wagner. Many of these wonderful people have used the opportunities that their CARESITES offered to reach out to others in need of help and have gone on to create foundations that can surely use your support. Please see these in *Ripples Go Forward* at the end of this guide.

I also want to thank Brooks Kenny and Courtney Allen of Lotsa Helping Hands for their enthusiastic embrace of this project and their interest in working together to help get this resource into the hands of families who truly need it.

I am similarly grateful to Russell Mark of the National Alliance for Caregiving for his wholehearted support of this project, including the wonderful list of resources included here and the Caregiver Self-Assessment Questionnaire that his organization developed for the American Medical Association.

Thank you's to Eugene Schwartz, Rabbi Goldie Milgram, Catherine Rehm, Andrew Bleckner, Livia Vanaver, Suzan Fine, Jamee Roberts and Tsurah August for critiquing this manuscript, and Naomi Hauser for her input on the transitions of care section. And to Susana Mayer for her marketing insights.

My gratitude also goes to Andrew Schorr for his passion for patient and family empowerment and, more specifically, inviting me to extend the reach of this guide with videos produced by his organization, Patient Power. Thanks also to Tamara Lobban-Jones for her video production expertise.

I want to thank my dear friend, Lenny Gerson, who made it his mission that I keep my eyes on the prize—my vision to create this series of guides and not get sidetracked by my other interests and passions. My gratitude continues to go out to my two long time mentors, Drs. Roger Bulger and Mack Lipkin, who continue to educate the medical provider community about care of people. And Gail Tuchman and Barbara Sarah for so many years of loving support.

And, of course, my dearest Tsurah, lover, joyful dance partner and co-life journeyer, whose love, support and wisdom mean everything to me. She continues to encourage me to passionately follow my dreams and live more and more consciously and kindly.

THE RIPPLES GO FORWARD

Foundations Created by and/or
Supported by Caresite Families

THE SARA'S SMILES FOUNDATION

www.saras-smiles.org

Created by the Burke family in memory of their daughter and granddaughter Sara.

Sara Burke was a vibrant, energetic, fun-loving, five year-old. She loved arts and crafts, mac 'n cheese, music, her Big Wheel, and her big brother and big sister. On May 12, 2008, Sara lost her courageous battle with cancer. The Sara's Smiles Foundation was created by Sara's family to carry on her memory, spirit and legacy of hope, determination and cheer. Sara's Smiles' mission is to help create smiles at a time when smiling may seem impossible by providing a variety of resources to entertain, comfort and educate children facing cancer and their families.

SMILES FROM ALI

www.smilesfromali.com

Created by Karen Borgen in memory of her daughter Lisa.

Smiles from Ali makes and sells entertaining items to raise money for childhood cancer research, and also donates them to children diagnosed with cancer (and their siblings) via pediatric units and the Rochester Ronald McDonald House.

LUNGEVITY FOUNDATION

http://events.lungevity.org

Supported by Mark Carlinsky in memory of his wife Lisa, who died of non-smoker related lung cancer.

The LUNGevity Foundation focuses on ensuring a higher quality of life and improving lung cancer survival rates by funding research into early detection and more effective treatment, as well as providing medically-expert education and support resources.

MOMMY'S LIGHT LIVES ON FUND

www.mommyslight.org

Supported by Mark Carlinsky in memory of his wife Lisa, and in honor of their son Matthew.

Mommy's Light helps children and teens with their grief process by celebrating a loved one's life through traditions they shared.

JANICE MCARDLE CANCER RESEARCH FOUNDATION

www.jannieshope.org

Supported by Mark Carlinsky.

The mission of the foundation is to fund innovative research to create awareness and education, develop early detection methods, advance treatment techniques, and ultimately find a cure for non-smoker related lung cancer.

LIAM'S LIGHTHOUSE FOUNDATION

http://www.liamslighthousefoundation.org

Created by Michelle Schulze in memory of her son Liam.

Liam's Lighthouse Foundation was established to create and provide educational material and awareness about Hemophagocytic Lymphohistiocytosis (HLH), including Histiocytic Disorders, and to distribute unbiased, factual information to physicians, hospitals and the community regarding this disease. The focus is also on bringing families affected by HLH/Histiocytosis together and offering support through a variety of resources, to raise funds for continued education to develop safer and more effective treatment methods and ultimately a cure, and to educate people about the importance of becoming a blood and bone marrow donor.

ABOUT THE AUTHOR

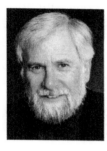 Yosaif August is a life coach, an award-winning healthcare innovator (Best of Competition, Nightingale Healthcare Design Awards, for inventing Bed-scapes®), an internationally published author, keynote speaker, and workshop presenter. *Coaching for Caregivers: How to Reach Out Before You Burn Out* is his second book and the first in a forthcoming series. His first book was *Help Me to Heal* (Hay House 2003), co-authored with Dr. Bernie Siegel.

Yosaif's life coaching practice, *Yes To Life Coaching*, has four areas of focus: *whole life, life transitions, health life*, and *coaching for caregivers*. With *whole life coaching*, Yosaif helps people attain greater fulfillment in their lives by seeing possibilities beyond their current sense of limitations and moving with passion and commitment towards those new possibilities. With *life transitions coaching*, he helps his clients use these transitions—career changes, retirement, relationships ending or beginning, parenting, starting new enterprises—as doorways to the lives they are truly meant to live. With *health life coaching*, he helps people with medical issues to manage their medical care while at the same time living their other parts of their lives to the fullest extent possible.

Yosaif also offers a private individualized *Coaching for Caregivers* program, utilizing the concepts and tools in this book. He helps caregivers feel their feet on the ground, assess their needs and develop a strategy for resiliently managing what they need to do.

His coaching repertoire includes using the creative arts—music, movement, visual arts, and humor—along with other techniques he has developed during his many years as an experiential educator. He encourages his clients to integrate their current spiritual and self-care practices into the coaching process. This enriches those practices and the coaching, as well.

His coaching is usually done via Skype, Facetime or Google Plus, and also via phone. This makes it especially accessible to people, i.e. caregivers, whose discretionary time is limited. He offers an initial complimentary session so that potential clients can experience his way of working and see how it might work for them.

For more information, see *http://www.yestolifecoaching.com*. To arrange a session, you can contact Yosaif at *august@yestolifecoaching.com*.

In his personal life, Yosaif loves to dance, sing and take nature walks with his wife; compose and play music; savor a good cup of coffee and enjoy food with his daughter; play bass to his son's lead guitar on Dylan and the Stones songs; make music, take "walk and talks," and play catch with his grandson; make his granddaughter fly; dote on his two cats; connect with friends close and far; and laugh with all of the above.

OTHER WORK BY YOSAIF AUGUST

Help Me to Heal
by Yosaif August and Bernie S. Siegel, M.D.
(Hay House 2003)

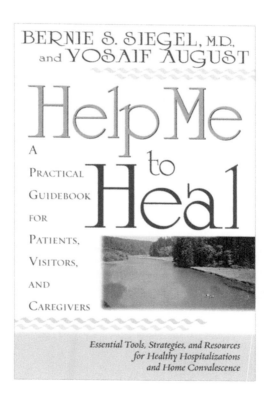

CarePages

Quick Tips Blog:
http://www.carepages.com/blogs/quicktips/posts

Hay House

Heal Your Life Blog:
http://www.healyourlife.com/search?q=yosaif

Yes To Life Coaching

Coaching for Caregivers Blog:
yestolifecoaching.com/caregivers/blog

CPSIA information can be obtained at www.ICGtesting.com
Printed in the USA
BVOW10s1056240813

329418BV00003B/9/P

9 780989 062619